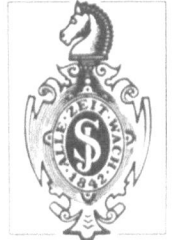

Springer-Verlag France
26, rue des Carmes, 75005 Paris

P. Diot, J.-L. Baulieu and E. Lemarié

Nuclear medicine and lung diseases

Prefaces by Pierre Jallet and Pierre Duroux

with 48 figures in black and white and 38 in colour

Springer-Verlag France S.A.R.L

Jean-Louis Baulieu, MD, PhD
Professor of Nuclear Medicine,
Department of Nuclear Medicine,
Centre Hospitalier Universitaire,
Tours, France

Patrice Diot, MD
Assistant,
Department of Respiratory Diseases and Physiology,
Centre Hospitalier Universitaire,
Tours, France

Etienne Lemarié, MD
Professor,
Department of Respiratory Diseases and Physiology,
Centre Hospitalier Universitaire,
Tours, France

Cover photograph: Perfusion scintigraphy with technetium-99m albumin macroaggregates, anterior view (Department of Nuclear Medicine, Centre Hospitalier et Universitaire, Tours).

© Springer-Verlag France 1993
Originally published by Springer-Verlag France, Paris in 1993.
Softcover reprint of the hardcover 1st edition 1993

ISBN 978-2-8178-0950-2   ISBN 978-2-8178-0948-9 (eBook)
DOI 10.1007/978-2-8178-0948-9

2918 / 3917 - 543210 / Printed on acid-free paper.

Table of contents

Contributors VII

Preface, Pierre Jallet 1

Preface, Pierre Duroux 3

Physical and technical bases, JL Baulieu 5
  Isotopes and radioactivity 5
    The atomic nucleus 5
    Radioactivity expression and units 7
    Parent-daughter decay 7
  Interaction between radiation and matter 7
    Absorption of charged particles 8
    Interactions and attenuation of photons 8
  Nuclear imaging 9
    Anger camera 9
    Data processing 10
  Radiopharmaceuticals 11
    The different forms of radio-pharmaceuticals 12

Physiopathological bases, P Diot and E Lemarié 13
  Structure of the respiratory tract 13
  Structure and function of the alveolo-capillary region 14
  Lung defense mechanisms 14
  Ventilation 15
    Disorders of lung ventilation 17
  Circulation 17
  Gas diffusion 17
  Ventilation-perfusion relationships 18
  Aerosols 18
    Aerosol properties 18
    Aerosol generators 20
    Mechanisms of aerosol deposition 20

Principles of the imaging process and analysis of images, S Bardet, F Baulieu, N Caillat-Vigneron,
S Coequyt, P Diot, J J Lafitte and P Peltier 23
   Perfusion scintigraphy 23
   Ventilation scintigraphy 24
      Radioactive gases 24
         Xenon-133 24
            Single breath technique 24
            Equilibration time method 24
         Krypton-81m 26
      Labeled aerosols 26
         Radioaerosol of technetium-99m Venticis™ 26
         Technegas™ 27
   Gallium scintigraphy 27
      Technical considerations 27
      Normal gallium-67 regional imaging 27
      Toxicity and dosimetry of gallium-67 29
         To assess hilar and mediastinal involvement in pulmonary malignancies 29
         To assesss extent and to follow up progression or response in the course
         of a lymphomatous disease 29
         To asses extent, location and inflammatory activity inflammatory activity of diffuse
         interstitial lung disease of disease of various origins 30
      Thoracic imaging with gallium-67 29
   DTPA scintigraphy 30
      Histological bases of DTPA clearance 31
      Physiology of the pulmonary clearance of technetium-99m DTPA 31
      Methods for study of the pulmonary clearance of technetium-99m DTPA 32
   Scintigraphy for the evaluation of mucociliary clearance 32
      Introduction 32
         The aerosol 33
         Production of the aerosol 33
         Image acquisition 33
      Image analysis 33
      Normal semiology 33
         Deposition index 33
         Presentation of results 34
         Data processing 34
      Pathologic semiology 34

Practical notions for carrying out nuclear medicine examination, JL Baulieu 39
   Referral and appointment 39
   Radioisotope availability and radiopharmaceutical preparation 39
   Tracer administration 40
   Imaging time 40
   Imaging support 41
   Interpretation - Report 42
   Act costing 42
   Irradiation - radioprotection 42
      Dosimetry - units 42
      Patient irradiation 43
      Radioprotection 43

Pulmonary embolism, F Baulieu and P Diot 45
   Place of isotopic techniques among diagnostic criteria 45

Radionuclide scanning techniques 47
    Perfusion scintigraphy 47
    Ventilation scintigraphy 49
        Gases 49
        Aerosols labeled with 99mTc 49
        Technegas™ 50
Interpretation of pulmonary scintigraphy and diagnostic strategy 50

Preoperative assessment of pulmonary function, F Baulieu and P Diot 53
Place of isotopic techniques 53
Imaging techniques 54
    Perfusion studies 54
    Ventilation studies 54
    Protocol example 55
Clinical relevance of lung scans 55

Diffuse interstitial lung diseases, P Diot , E Lemarié, A Le Pape, P Peltier and N Caillat-Vigneron 57
Current concepts 57
    Pathogenesis: alveolitis and fibrosis 57
    Diffuse interstitial lung disease from the perspective of the clinician 58
    Markers of activity 60
Radionuclide scanning techniques 61
    Gallium-67 scanning 61
        Mechanisms of gallium-67 accumulation in inflammatory lesions 61
        Pulmonary sarcoidosis 61
        Histiocytosis X 65
        Wegener's granulomatosis 66
        Pulmonary infiltrates with eosinophilia 66
        Idiopathic pulmonary fibrosis or usual interstitial pneumonia (UIP) 67
        Interstitial lung disease associated with connective tissue diseases 67
        Diffuse interstitial lung diseases with known etiologies 70
            Pneumoconioses 70
            Hypersensitivity pneumonitis 71
    Macrophage scintigraphy 72
    99mTc-DTPA scintigraphy 75

Lung tumors, JL Baulieu, P Bourguet, B Desrues and E Lemarié 79
Introduction 79
Nuclear medicine procedures for tumor-localisation 80
    Immunoscintigraphy 80
        Monoclonal antibodies and their labeling 80
        Tumor associated antigens 80
        Immunoscintigraphy in lung cancer 81
    Gallium scintigraphy 82
    Macrophage scintigraphy 84
    SMS and MIBG scintigraphy 85
        MIBG scintigraphy 85
        SMS scintigraphy 86

Infectious diseases, A Moisan and ML Quinquenel 89
Methods 89
    Gallium-67 scintigraphy (67Ga) 89

Labeled leukocyte scintigraphy 89
    In vitro labeling procedure 89
        Indium-111 90
        Technetium-99m (^{99m}Tc) 90
        Results 90
    In vivo labeling procedure 90
Human non-specific polyclonal immunoglobulin scintigraphy 91
Indications and perspectives of scintigraphy 91
Conclusion 92

Radionuclide imaging in pulmonary complications of Human Immunodeficiency Virus infection,
J Cadranel, J Rosso, C Mayaud and M Meignan 95
Gallium lung scanning in HIV infected patients 95
Background 95
Results of gallium lung scanning in AIDS patients with suspected pneumocystis carinii pneumonia 96
    Specificity and sensitivity 96
    Value of gallium scanning follow-up after therapy for PCP 97
    Mechanism of gallium uptake in PCP 98
Results of gallium lung scanning in AIDS patients free from pneumocystis carinii pneumonia 98
    Results of gallium scan in non-PCP infections 99
    Results of gallium scan in HIV-associated lymphoid processes 99
    Results of gallium scan in pulmonary Kaposi sarcoma 99
    Comparison between gallium and indium-111-labeled autologous leukocyte lung scans 99
Value of whole body gallium scanning in pulmonary complications of HIV infection 99
Guidelines for the use of gallium lung scanning in HIV seropositive patients 100
Tc-DTPA lung scanning in HIV infected patients 100
Background 100
Assessment of pulmonary epithelial permeability in pulmonary complications of HIV infection 101
    Pulmonary epithelial permeability in HIV associated lymphocytic alveolitis 101
    Pulmonary epithelial permeability in PCP 101
Comparison of gallium lung scan and Tc-DTPA clearance in pulmonary complications
of HIV infection 101
Are there recommendations for the use of Tc-DTPA scanning in HIV seropositive patients? 103
Conclusion 104

Chronic obstructive pulmonary diseases, F Baulieu, S Coequyt and JJ Laffitte 107
Mucociliary clearance 107
Mucociliary escalator 107
Methods for the evaluation of mucociliary clearance 107
Mucociliary clearance study in clinical practice 108
    Diagnostic value of mucociliary clearance study 108
    Evaluation of pharmacological agents on lung mucociliary clearance 108
Gastro-esophageal scintigraphy 108
Scintigraphic procedure 109

Right to left shunt, JL Baulieu 111

Nuclear Medicine and the pediatric lung, D Poncin, F Bonnin and B Bok 113
Specific problems in children 113
Radiation doses in children 113
Methods 113
Ventilation studies 113

    Perfusion studies 114
    Nuclear medicine (pulmonary) procedures in children 114
    Scintigraphic maturation patterns 114
  Scintigraphic imaging in pediatric pulmonary pathology 114
    Foreign body inhalation 114
    Primary bronchiectasis and sequelae of infectious disease 115
    Pulmonary embolism 115
    Congenital lung and heart abnormalities 115
    Asthma 115
    Mucoviscidosis 115
    Chest tumors 115
    Scoliosis 115
    Recurrent chest disease and gastro-esophageal reflux 115
  Conclusion 116

Optimization of aerosol therapy by nuclear medicine techniques, P Diot and G Smaldone 117
  Methodology 117
  Applications 119

Index 123

Contributors

Stéphane Bardet, MD
Assistant, Department of Nuclear Medicine, Centre Hospitalier Universitaire, Nantes, Hôtel Dieu, France

Françoise Baulieu, MD
Nuclear Physician, Department of Nuclear Medicine, Centre Hospitalier Universitaire, Tours, France

Jean-Louis Baulieu, MD, PhD
Professor of Nuclear Medicine, Department of Nuclear Medicine, Centre Hospitalier Universitaire, Tours, France

Bernard Bok, MD, PhD
Professor of Nuclear Medicine, Department of Nuclear Medicine, Centre Hospitalier Universitaire Beaujon, Clichy, France

François Bonnln, MD
Assistant, Department of Nuclear Medicine, Centre Hospitalier Universitaire Beaujon, Clichy, France

Patrick Bourguet, MD, PhD
Professor of Nuclear Medicine, Department of Nuclear Medicine, Centre Hospitalier Universitaire, Rennes, France

Jacques Cadranel, MD
Department of Pulmonary Diseases, Hopital Tenon, Paris, France

Nadine Caillat-Vigneron, MD
Nuclear Physician, Service Central de Médecine Nucléaire et de Biophysique, Hopital Avicenne, Bobigny, France

Serge Coequyt, MD
Nuclear Physician, Service Central de Médecine Nucléaire, Centre Hospitalier Régional et Universitaire de Lille, France

Benoit Desrues, MD
Department of Pulmonary Disease, Centre Hospitalier Universitaire, Rennes, France

Patrice Diot, MD
Assistant, Department of Respiratory Diseases and Physiology, Centre Hospitalier Universitaire, Tours, France

Jean-Jacques Laffite, MD
Professor, Departement de Pneumologie, Centre Hospitalier Régional et Universitaire de Lille, France

Etienne Lemarié, MD
Professor, Department of Respiratory Diseases and Physiology, Centre Hospitalier Universitaire, Tours, France

Alain Le Pape, PhD
Director, Laboratoire de Biophysique Cellulaire, Inserm U316, Faculté de Médecine de Tours, France

Charles Mayaud, MD
Professor, Department of Respiratory Diseases, Hopital Tenon, Paris, France

Michel Meignan, MD, PhD
Professor of Nuclear Medicine, Department of Nuclear Medicine,
Centre Hospitalier Universitaire Henri Mondor, Créteil, France

Annick Moisan, MD
Assistant, Centre Régional de Lutte Contre le Cancer, Hôpital Pontchaillou, Rennes, France

Patrick Peltier, MD, PhD
Department of Nuclear Medicine, Centre Hospitalier Universitaire, Nantes, Hôtel Dieu, France

Didier Poncin, MD
Assistant, Department of Nuclear Medicine, Centre Hospitalier Universitaire Beaujon, Clichy, France

Marie-Line Quinquenel, MD
Assistant, Department of Pulmonary Diseases, Centre Hospitalier Universitaire, Rennes, France

Jean Rosso, MD
Assistant, Department of Nuclear Medicine, Centre Hospitalier Universitaire Henri Mondor, Créteil, France

Gerald Smaldone, MD, PhD
Associate Professor of Medicine, Physiology and Biophysics, Health Sciences Center, State University of New York at Stony Brook, NY, USA

Preface

Among the various examinations performed in most Nuclear Medicine Departments, lung scintigraphy is the third most common after bone and heart scintigraphy. However few recent books present the current situation concerning lung scintigraphy or allow clinicians or nuclear physicians to exploit fully the possibilities offered by this isotopic examination. Perfusion scintigraphy is commonly accepted for the diagnosis of pulmonary embolism, however a standardized method has yet to be defined for quantitating perfusion defects, and the role of ventilation scintigraphy is still under discussion.

Three-dimensional and dynamic imaging are routine for functional studies of many organs with nuclear imaging. What is the situation with dynamic and tomographic lung imaging? Sophisticated imaging processes have been made available by the manufacturers of imaging systems. And what about image processing and quantification in the investigation of pulmonary function? Many new radiolabeled molecules have been proposed as optimal function investigation agents and specific lesion markers. What is the situation with the development of new functional exploration methods on the basis of these new radiopharmaceutical products?

These questions were the background of the collaboration between clinicians and nuclear physicians which resulted in this book.

The book has three aims:

The first aim is to revise the elements of both Nuclear Medecine technology and lung physio-pathology, the bases of functional imaging. The first three chapters are particularly concerned with this. The authors have chosen to give a practical guide based on their experience rather than an exhaustive review of the literature.

The second aim is to present the new methods based on recently developed radiopharmaceutical agents such as agents for ventilation study, metabolic markers, particularly amine uptake markers and tumor markers such as antibodies, somatostatin receptor ligands and activated macrophage markers.

The third aim is to describe the use of scintigraphic information in actual clinical situations: in pre-operative evaluation, in the acquired immuno-deficiency syndrome and in aerosol therapy.

This book gives valuable aid on these subjects to pneumologists and nuclear physicians as well as to experienced practitioners and students wishing to specialize. Readers will judge whether the authors have succeeded. Their judgement should strongly encourage the publishing of other books written with the same spirit of collaboration between clinicians and nuclear physicians in other spheres of Nuclear Medicine.

Pierre Jallet
President of the Société Française de Biophysique
et Médecine Nucléaire

Preface

Treatment of patients with pulmonary disease begins with the consultation interview followed by the physical examination. Additional examinations guide treatment or confirm diagnosis. Pulmonary scintigraphy, bronchofibroscopy and pulmonary function tests (PFTs) are among the additional examinations available.

Radioisotopes are commonly used in pneumology. On the one hand, on the basis of PFT data and lung perfusion scintigraphy, they are used in the pre-operative evaluation of primary bronchial carcinomas in order to predict post-operative ventilation. On the other hand, they are used for diagnosis and for follow-up of treatment and evolution of acute pulmonary embolism and vascular lung disease generally.

Routine use of radioisotopes is not without problems if we wish to obtain regularly good quality pulmonary scintigrams in the first hours or days after the appearance of initial symptoms which can finally be correctly interpreted in terms of clinical and radiological data (pulmonary or pleural opacity).

Readers of this book will find in this high quality, clear and well-documented text, anatomical, physiological and biophysical bases which make possible better understanding and use of complementary examinations such as pulmonary scintigraphy which they use every day. Reading this book will show them that technical progress will occur in the future, particularly in the definition and quantification of radioisotope images.

It will be necessary to plan an increase in the indications for radioisotopes in lung disease, in particular for the detection of metastases in primary lung cancer and for the treatment of AIDS patients with respiratory conditions. The validation of experimental studies of radioisotopes and their application to clinical use will certainly, and very soon, change the treatment of such fundamental and frequent diseases as AIDS and primary bronchial carcinoma.

Pierre Duroux
Vice-President of the Société de Pneumologie
de Langue Française

Physical and technical bases

JL Baulieu

Isotopes and radio-activity

The atomic nucleus

The atomic nucleus is comprised of protons and neutrons which are known as nucleons. The protons have a positive electrical charge.The neutrons have no electrical charge. The number of protons determines the atomic number of the atom (Z). This determines also the number of orbital electrons and therefore the chemical element to which the atom belongs.

The total number of nucleons is the mass number (A) of the nucleus. The difference (A-Z) is the neutron number (N).

The nuclei with the same proton number and different mass number are called isotopes. They have the same chemical properties but different nuclear properties. Some are stable and some are not stable, due either to a relative excess of neutrons or a relative excess of protons. On a graph N / Z, the stable nuclides are clustered around an imaging line called the line of stability (N ≈ Z for light elements, N ≈ 1.5.Z for heavy elements) (fig. 1). An unstable nucleus transforms into a more stable nucleus. This is the process of radioactive disintegration or radioactive decay.

The nuclei with a relative excess of neutrons are ß⁻ emitters: a neutron in the nucleus is transformed into a proton and an electron:

$$n \rightarrow p^+ + e^- + \bar{v} + \text{energy}$$

The electron (e⁻) and the anti-neutrino ($\bar{v}$) are ejected from the nucleus. The electron is called a beta particle. The energy released is shared between the ß⁻ particle and the anti-neutrino.

Decay results in a transmutation. The parent radionuclide (X) and daughter product (Y) represent different chemical elements because their atomic number Z is different. It increases by one:

$$^A_Z X \xrightarrow{\beta^-} \; ^A_{Z+1} Y$$

Most often, the ß⁻ decay is accompanied by a γ emission because the daughter nuclide is produced in an excited state, which immediately returns to the stable state.

Example: xenon-133

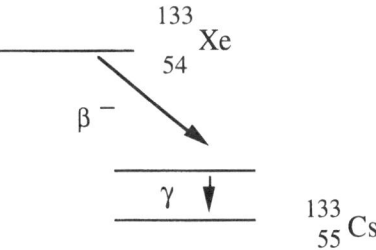

In other cases, the ß⁻ decay results in a metastable excited state. This means that the daughter nucleus decays with delay to a more stable nuclear arrangement by the emission of a γ photon:

$$^A_Z X \xrightarrow{\beta^-} \; ^A_{Z+1} Y^* \xrightarrow{\gamma} \; ^A_{Z+1} Y$$

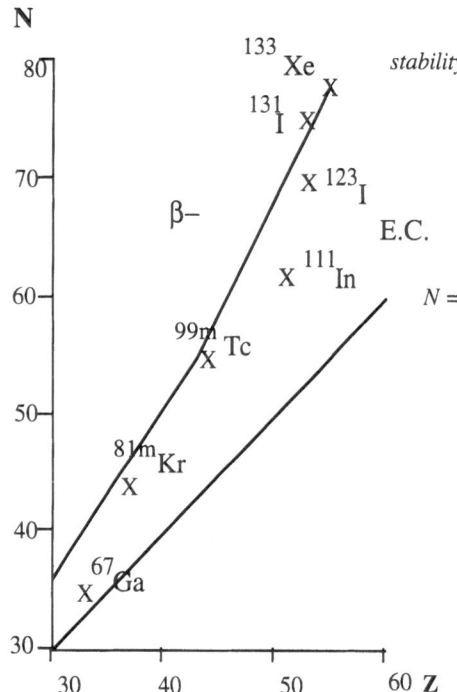

Fig. 1. Nucleon distribution in some radio-nuclides. Z = number of protons, N = number of neutrons. The radio-nuclides with an excess of neutrons (^{133}Xe, ^{131}I) are on the left of the stability line and are beta-emitters (ß⁻). The radio-nuclides with an excess of protons (^{123}I, ^{111}In, ^{67}Ga) are on the right of the stability line and decay by electronic capture (E.C.). The radio-nuclides located on the stability line (^{99m}Tc, ^{81m}Kr) decay by isomeric transition

Example: technetium-99m

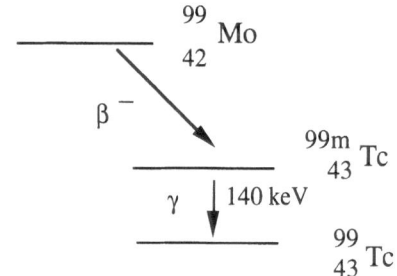

The nuclei with a relative excess of protons decay by ß⁺ emission or by electronic capture.

In ß⁺ emission, a proton in the nucleus is transformed into a neutron and a positively charged electron called positon:

$$p^+ \rightarrow n + e^+ + \nu + energy$$

The positon and the neutrino are ejected from the nucleus. The positon loses its kinetic energy in collisions with atoms of the surrounding matter and comes to rest, usually within a few millimeters of the site of its origin. The positon then combines with an ordinary electron in an annihilation reaction: the mass of the particles is converted into energy. The mass-energy equivalent of each particle is 0.511 MeV. This energy appears in the form of two 0.511 MeV annihilation photons, which are emitted in exactly opposite directions (180° apart). Thus, decay by ß⁺ emission ultimately results in the production of two 0.511 MeV photons:

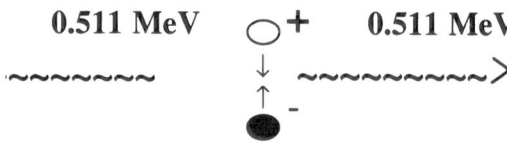

The decay results in a transmutation: the atomic number decreases by one:

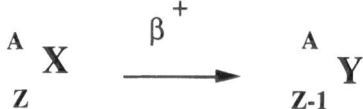

Example: oxygen 15

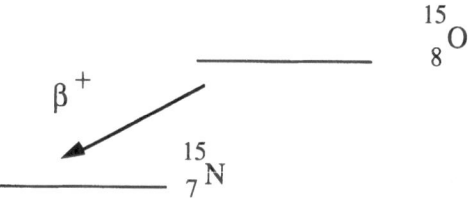

In electron capture, an orbital electron is captured by the nucleus and combines with a proton to form a neutron:

$$p^+ + e^- \rightarrow n + \nu + energy$$

As in ß+ decay the atomic number decreases by one:

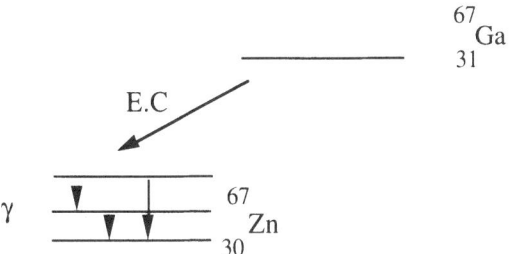

Example: gallium-67

To summarize schematically, two types of radiation are emitted during radioactive transformations:

– ß⁻ particles – corpuscular and charged radiation,

– γ photons – electro-magnetic radiation,

–X rays are also emitted following the rearrangement of electronic orbitals of the atom, especially after electronic capture.

Radioactivity expression and units

In a sample containing N atoms of one radionuclide, the probability of one atom undergoing radioactive decay in the time unit is given by λ, the decay constant of the radionuclide. The decay constant is a characteristic constant of each radionuclide. During the period of time dt, the number of atoms which decay is:

$dN = - \lambda N dt$ (1)

The unit of λ is [time]⁻¹. The minus sign indicates that dN decreases with time. The quantity λ.N is the activity of the sample:

$A = \lambda.N$ (2)

The legal international unit of activity is the becquerel (Bq). A sample which has a 1 Bq activity means that it decays at a rate of 1 sec⁻¹ (one disintegration per second). Multiples of the becquerel are the kilobecquerel (1 kBq = 10^3 Bq), megabecquerel (1 MBq = 10^6 Bq), and the gigabecquerel (1 GBq = 10^9 Bq).

However, the traditional unit is the curie (Ci), which is still commonly used in day-to-day practice. The curie was originally defined as the activity of 1 gram of ^{226}Ra (radium) i.e, $3.7 . 10^{10}$ disintegrations per second:

$1 Ci = 3.7 . 10^{10}$ Bq.

This represents a relatively high radioactivity. The submultiples of the curie are the millicurie (1mCi = 10^{-3} Ci) and the microcurie (1µCi = 10^{-6} Ci).

The amount of radioactivity used for nuclear medicine studies typically are in the 50 µCi – 20 mCi, 2 MBq – 800 MBq range.

From the above equations (1) and (2), it can be calculated that:

$N(t) = N(0) . e^{-\lambda t}$

and

$A(t) = A(0) . e^{-\lambda t}$

Therefore, the number of radioactive atoms and the activity remaining in the sample decrease with time according to an exponential law. Exponential decay is characterized by the disappearance of a constant fraction of activity or number of atoms per time unit. A constant fraction of the radioactivity present in the sample disappears during a given time interval. The half-life (T) of a radionuclide is the time required for it to decay to 50% of its initial activity level. On a semilogarithmic (arithmetic scale on the horizontal axis, logarithmic scale on the vertical axis), the time activity curve is represented by a straight line (fig. 2). The decay constant λ and the half-life T are characteristic for a specific radionuclide. Their values are listed in a table which is called a radionuclide chart. The two constants are related by the equation:

$$\lambda = \frac{Log2}{T} = \frac{0,693}{T}$$

Parent-daughter decay

A particular situation occurs when a sample contains two radionuclides having a parent-daughter relationship. The daughter product is being formed at the time it is decaying. When the parent half-life is longer than the daughter half-life, the daughter activity in the sample increases, reaches a maximum and then decreases following the decay of the parent. The parent and the daughter are said to be in transient equilibrium. An example is the ^{99}Mo to ^{99m}Tc decay:

^{99}Mo (T = 66 hr) T ^{99m}Tc (T = 6 hr)

Interaction between radiation and matter

The passage of radiation through matter causes ionisation (removal of one or several electrons from the atoms in the matter) and excitation (change of energy level of one or several electrons in the atom). By these mechanisms, the energy of the radiation is transferred to the matter. The corpuscular charged

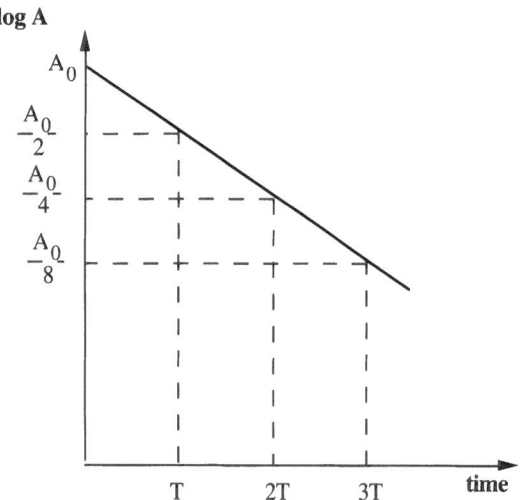

Fig. 2. Radio-active decay of one radio-nuclide. Radio-activity (A) decreases by a factor of 2 during each period of time, equal to T, the physical half-life of the nuclide. The time-activity curve is a straight line in a semi-logarithmic plot.

radiations (ß⁻ and ß⁺) are directly ionizing radiations. The electromagnetic radiations (γ) are indirectly ionizing radiations. Ionization and excitation are the underlying mechanisms for most radiation detectors and radiobiological effects.

Absorption of charged particles

The collisions of charged particles with the atomic electrons creates ionized and excited atoms: the charged particles are directly ionizing radiations.

The distance travelled in the matter, or range, of the electrons generated by ß⁻ emission depends on the energy of the electrons and on the density of the absorbing material. The maximum range in water expressed in cm is about equal to half of the maximum energy ($E_{ßmax}$) expressed in MeV, and is inversely proportional to the density of the absorbing material. For example, the range of the electron beams emitted by ^{133}Xe (xenon, $E_{ßmax} = 0.1$ MeV) is 0.05 cm in water and 39 cm in air. The ß⁻ radiation beam emitted by an internal radionuclide is completely absorbed in the body. It is responsible for most of the irradiation dose delivered to the body, and does not contribute to the external detection.

Interactions and attenuation of photons

The γ photons interact in the matter according mainly to two modalities: the photoelectric and the Compton effects.

The photoelectric effect is an atomic absorption process in which an atom totally absorbs the energy of a photon. The photon disappears and its energy is used to eject an orbital electron from the atom. The ejected electron is called a photoelectron and interacts forwards in the matter as a charged particle. Photons are indirectly ionizing radiations.

In some materials, a portion of the energy is released as visible light. These materials are called scintillators. Most radiation detectors are made of scintillators and are called scintillation detectors (see paragraph "Anger camera"). As the energy of the photon is fully deposited in the material, the scintillation intensity is proportional to the photon energy. A single radioisotope in the source provides a single peak on an amplitude signal spectrum obtained by the scintillation detector. This peak is called the photopeak. The photopeak energy is characteristic of the radioisotope.

Compton scattering is a collision between a photon and a free electron. The photon energy is partially transferred to the electron. The photon is deflected through a scattering angle. The consequence is the emission of secondary photons out of the source and a broad band on the amplitude signal spectrum. The scattered photons blur the image obtained through scintillation imaging systems. They must be eliminated; this is possible by energy discrimination techniques (see paragraph "Anger camera").

Other interactions such as pair production (photon materialisation in e⁻ and e⁺) can occur. However they occur at high photon energy more than 1 MeV. Therefore, they are of little practical importance with commonly used radioelements the energy of which is from 80 to 364 keV.

The probability that a photon will experience an interaction is inversely proportional to its energy and depends on the composition and the thickness of the absorbing material. The attenuation of the photon beam is a decreasing exponential function of the

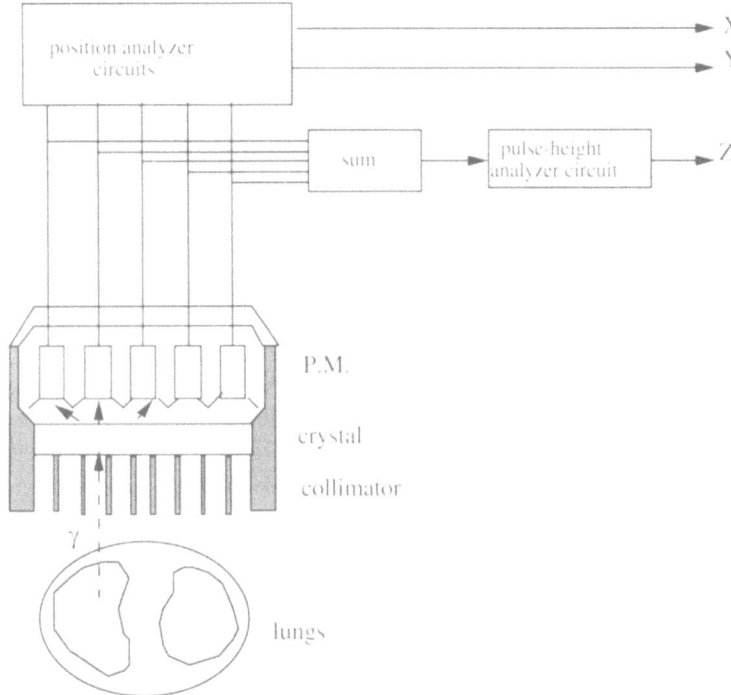

Fig.3. Schematic representation of the Anger gamma-camera

absorber thickness. Usually, the γ radiation beam emitted by an internal radionuclide in the body is attenuated, not absorbed. The contribution of γ emission to the irradiation dose is low. It makes possible external detection and imaging.

Nuclear imaging

Anger camera

The scintillation gamma camera was developed by H. Anger in 1953. It has become the standard nuclear imaging instrument for clinical applications.

The general concept is the detection of the scintillations produced by the interaction of a γ ray in a large scintillator crystal (see paragraph "Interaction and attenuation of protons").

The crystal is composed of sodium iodide containing traces of thallium impurities, NaI(Tl). The crystal is circular or rectangular 30 to 50 cm wide x 1.2 cm thick. The side of the crystal facing the γ ray beam is covered by the collimator.

The collimator comprises lead septa separating holes. The direction of the holes, most often parallel, selects the direction of the γ ray which will reach the crystal. Thus, the γ rays are projected from the source distribution onto the crystal surface. The distribution of the scintillations in the crystal outlines the

distribution of the radioactivity in front of the crystal. The signal of each scintillation is amplified and positioned by a photomultiplier (PM) tube array viewing the rear surface of the crystal.

Electronic position analysis circuits connected to the PM determine the location of each scintillation event as it occurs in the crystal. The signal is also analyzed for energy by the pulse-height analyzer circuit.

In conclusion, each γ ray detected by the camera generates 3 signals:
- x, y coordinates for position,
- z for pulse height i.e. energy (fig. 3).

At the present time, the gamma camera works according to various imaging modalities:

Static imaging — the steady radionuclide distribution is imaged over an extended imaging time, e.g. lung distribution of labeled microspheres for perfusion studies,

Dynamic imaging — time evolution of the radionuclide distribution is followed by a temporal sequence on a digital image storage system, e.g. wash in and wash out of xenon for ventilation studies,

Tomographic imaging — the three dimensional distribution of the radioactivity is recorded by rotation of the camera over 180° or 360° around the source organ, and the computer proceeds to the reconstruction of cross-sectional images along different plane orientations, e.g. improvement of small perfusion defect detection,

Whole body imaging — the camera scans the body linearly from head to feet allowing imaging of the whole body. This modality is used for detection of malignant bone tumor metastases.

One interesting equipment option is the double head camera: this device allows a decrease in patient examination time and an increase in the number of detected events and therefore improvement of the image quality.

Despite continuous technical improvements during last three decades, the Anger camera performance suffers from limitations in terms of image uniformity, spatial resolution, detection sensitivity and counting linearity.

Image non-uniformity is assessed by exposing the detector crystal to a uniform flux of radiation. The produced images present small but noticeable variations in intensity, even with a properly functioning camera. These variations may be equivalent to counting rate variations of ±10% or more. Image non-uniformity is maintained at the lowest level by precise calibration and repeated controls of pulse-height spectra for each PM tube and electronic position analyser circuits.

Spatial resolution is the minimal distance between two sources that can be distinctly perceived. It is usually about 8–12 cm. The resolution is limited by the material itself, i.e. crystal thickness and collimator hole diameter and also by the detection conditions. Two are especially important:

The energy window, strict fitting with the photopeak and width close to 15% of the energy of the photopeak, in order to reduce blurring due to scattered photons.

Position of the patient as near as possible to the collimator.

Detection efficiency mainly depends on the crystal thickness and collimator hole diameter. Increasing the crystal thickness and collimator hole diameter improves detection efficiency but impairs spatial resolution. Thus a compromise has to be found between sensitivity and resolution which differs according to the purpose of the examination. Usually, resolution is favored in static and tomographic imaging, for example in perfusion studies; efficiency is favored in dynamic studies using low tracer activity such as xenon ventilation studies.

Counting linearity becomes questionable at high counting rates. The camera behaves as a paralyzable system and the counting loss is proportional to the dead time, the minimal time between two consecutive events which can be separately detected.

Usually, the dead time is about 10 μsec and counting losses become consistent for a counting rate of 10^4 counts per second. Deadtime losses are typically a problem in the first-pass cardiac flow studies but are generally not involved in most lung studies.

Data processing

Since about 1985, the cameras have been numeric or digital. The analogic x, y, z signals are converted into bits at the detector output.

The scintigraphic images are displayed on a 64x64, 128x128 or 256x256 pixel (picture element) matrix. The choice of the matrix size depends on the spatial resolution R and on the field of view of the camera. The pixel size must be less than R/2. Considering a 10mm resolution and 400mm diameter field of view camera, the pixel size must be less than 10 mm/2 = 5 mm/pixel and the matrix size more than 400 mm/ 5mm = 80 pixels, i.e. in practice 128x128 pixels.

One of the advantages of numeric cameras is that detector performances are under the control of a microprocessor and can be automatically optimized. For example, non-uniformity is corrected using a test image of a uniform radiation field. For each radioelement, a matrix of correction factors is generated from the uniform radiation field acquisition, stored in the data processing system memory, and used for the correction of matrices acquired subsequently.

The processing of static images includes displaying and quantification. The value of each pixel, the number of disintegrations recorded at the pixel coordinates x, y, is coded by a gray or colour scale. Usually, the value of each pixel is coded by 8 bits. Therefore, the theoretical number of gray levels or colours is $2^8 = 256$. In practice, the gray scale includes only 40 levels which is the maximal number that the human eye can distinguish. The colour scale provides a broader range of coding colours. However, the colour display can produce image artefacts such as pseudo-contours due to apparently sharp changes in pixel values where none actually exist. For this reason, the colour scale must always be displayed associated with the digital image.

When a high activity spot is present in an image it can be useful to mask the region of the hot spot, or to attribute the maximum gray or colour level to a pixel value inferior to the maximal activity. By this procedure, the colour scale is spread out in the range of relevant activity and allows a better analysis of the image. For example, mouth activity due to aerosol stagnation impairs the vizualization of lower lung activity. This can be corrected by appropriate masking or scaling.

Quantitative information is extracted from the matrix image by displaying the count in one pixel or in a set of pixels present in a region of interest (ROI). The count in a pixel or in a ROI does not exactly measure the source object radioactivity. Many factors affect the measurement of radioactivity by the camera. The most important are attenuation and diffusion of the radiation beam and partial volume effect. The partial volume effect is the modification of source count due to the size of the source: small objects near the resolution value appear to contain smaller concentrations of radioactivity than they actually do. Thus, it is more precise to perform quantitative analysis by using the count ratio or index than absolute radioactivity measurement.

The data processing systems are especially powerful in processing image sequences according to time, space or energy.

A temporal image sequence contains information about the tracer kinetics. Time activity curves are generated from each lung or from a part of the lung. The operator has to draw and position ROI's.

The computer calculates and generates time-activity curves. The curves can be fitted to a mathematical function such as mono or multi-exponential function. It is possible to calculate kinetic parameters such as biological period or clearance. These methods are useful for ventilation, mucociliary function or alveolo-capillary permeability studies.

A spatial sequence is obtained by a 360° or 180° camera rotation. For example 64 subsequent images are recorded during rotation. The sequence of the bidimensional projection images contains the information related to the three-dimensional activity distribution. This information is processed and displayed as bidimensional matrices in transverse, sagittal and frontal planes.

The usual reconstruction method is the filtered backprojection algorithm. Each line of recorded matrices represents an activity profile which is expanded along the incident direction giving a backprojection. Superimposition of backprojections obtained from a rotation results in a cross-sectional image of the object. The procedure is repeated for each line and thus the tomographic imaging of the scintigraphic object is obtained. Reconstruction processing creates noise in the images which is reduced by appropriate filtering. Tomographic

acquisition requires stable activity distribution. It is feasible for perfusion studies by radiolabeled tracer embolization.

A sequence of different energy images is obtained by simultaneous or consecutive acquisitions of different isotopes with a different energy. The energy discrimination is performed by the pulse-height analyser. When an isotope produces γ photons with several energies, the pulse height analyser allows the recording of each γ photo-peak.

Radiopharmaceuticals

The radioelements used in lung scintigraphy are presented in table 1, with their physical properties and radiopharmaceutical presentation.

The favorable ^{99m}Tc half-life (T = 6hr) and γ energy explain its wide use especially for perfusion studies with macroaggregates and microspheres. ^{99m}Tc is available from a generator containing the parent element: ^{99}Mo. The generator activity decreases with the parent half-life (T = 66hr) because parent and daughter are in transient equilibrium (see paragraph "Parent-daughter decay"). Thus, the generator is used for 5 to 7 days and changed once or twice the week. The cost of a generator varies according to its activity (1,850 MBq to 18,500 MBq) from 1,730 FF to 5,550 FF (december 92).

Some radioelements (^{131}I, ^{133}Xe) are fission products. They are available from a nuclear reactor. Their price is relatively low.

Other radioelements (^{67}Ga, ^{111}In) are produced in other nuclear reactions involving accelerated particles generated in an accelerator such as a cyclotron. The disposal of these elements is less immediate and their cost is higher.

The physical half-life is a practical limiting factor. ^{81m}Kr has a very short half-life (T = 13 sec) and can be used only from a generator in transient equilibrium with its parent: ^{81}Rb (T = 4.6 hr). On the other hand, relatively long half-life elements such as ^{131}I can be stored some days before use. However they raise the problem of irradiation dose and radioprotection (see chapter "Practical notions for carrying out nuclear medicine examination").

^{131}I, which is a β^- emitter, is a therapeutic agent of differentiated thyroid cancer metastases in the lung. The therapeutic activity is about 7 GBq. This treatment requires a 5 to 7 day stay in a room with urine collection in a decontamination tank.

When a radioelement has a γ emission with several energies (^{67}Ga, ^{111}In) the different photopeaks can be

Table 1. γ-emitters used in lung scintigraphy

Radioisotope	Symbol	Physical half-life	Radiation	Production	Radiopharma-ceutical form	Application	Cost FF/dose
Technetium-99m metastable	^{99m}Tc	6 hr	γ 140 keV	Generator	Macroaggegates Microspheres Aerosol Sulfocolloid Glycopeptide Phosphonate	Perfusion " Ventilation Esophagal transit Inflammation Bone scan	1420 1740 780 1030
Iodine-123	^{123}I	13.3 hr	γ 159 keV	Cyclotron	MIBG[1] solution IAMP[2] " SMS[3] "	Monoamine uptake " Tumor labelling	1370 1370
Iodine-131	^{131}I	8.1 j	β⁻ γ 364 keV	Reactor	Iodide solution	Thyroid cancer Metastases	420
Xenon-133	^{133}Xe	5.3 j	β⁻ γ 81 keV	Reactor	Gas	Ventilation Perfusion	800
Krypton-81m	^{81m}Kr	13 sec	γ 190 keV	Generator	Gas	Ventilation	
Gallium-67	^{67}Ga	78 hr	γ 93 keV 184 keV 296 keV	Cyclotron	Gallium citrate Solution	Inflammation Tumor	1580
Indium -111	^{111}In	2.8 j	γ 172keV 247 keV	Cyclotron	Antibodies, SMS[3] Polynuclears Platelets	Tumor Infection	950

[1] MIBG = meta-iodobenzylguanidine, [2] IAMP = iodoamphétamine, [3] SMS = somatostatine octreodide analog

detected and added (see paragraph "Data processing"). This increases detection sensitivity.

However, the image quality can possibly be altered by Compton diffusion and by the transparency of the collimator's septa for high energy photons. Therefore, spectrometry has to be carefully adjusted and a medium or high energy collimator used.

The different forms of radiopharmaceuticals

– Solid particle or cell suspension in a liquid phase: macroaggregates, microspheres, sulfocolloid, polynuclears, platelets;
    – solid particles in a gasous phase: aerosol;

– gas: xenon, krypton;

– atomic or molecular solution: iodide, gallium, meta-iodo benzylguanidine (MIBG), iodoamphetamine (IAMP), somatostatine analog octreotide (SMS), antibodies.

The three first classes are the most useful for functional investigation of the lung. The atomic or molecular solutions are cell markers.They are not yet largely used in pneumology but their development is in progress.

Reference

1. Sorenson JA, Phelps ME (1987) Physics in Nuclear Medicine (2nd edition) Grune and Straton

Physiopathological bases

P Diot and E Lemarié

Imaging procedures such as X-ray, ultrasound, computed tomography and magnetic resonance express differences in density. Diagnostic information obtained by nuclear medicine is based on differences in concentration of radiolabeled tracers. This concentration depends on the characteristics of the tracer and the physiological conditions. Thus, nuclear imaging expresses functional characteristics of the respiratory system and is complementary to the anatomic imaging. Therefore it is necessary to understand the bases of respiratory physiology to explain images obtained with radiolabeled tracers.

Structure of the respiratory tract

The bronchopulmonary system comprises two lungs and the airways. The right lung accounts for 55% of total lung function. The right lung consists of 3 lobes, upper, middle and lower. The left lung has only two lobes, upper and lower. The upper lobe comprises two segments, an upper division comparable to the right upper lobe and a lower, lingular division, comparable to the right middle lobe.

The airways are arranged in generations and the number and total diameters increase from the trachea to the small airways (fig. 1). Where the airways become narrower, they become more numerous, so that the total cross-sectional area increases. The conductive zone of the tracheobronchial tree begins at the trachea under the larynx. The larynx is the narrowest part of the airway. The trachea is 15 to 20 mm in diameter and the terminal bronchiole is 0.5 mm in diameter. The trachea is divided into 2 main bronchi (generation 1), lobar bronchi (generation 2) and finishes with the terminal bronchiole (generations 14-15). The respiratory zone comprises respiratory bronchioles (generations 15-16), the alveolar duct, the alveolar sac and finally the alveolus (generations 23-24). At the other end, the alveolar surface reaches an area of 70 to 80 m^2. The consequence is a decrease in resistance to air flow from the larynx and trachea to the alveoli. The resistance to air flow is due to the larynx (50%), from the trachea to the small bronchi (40%) and the peripheral airways (10%). These data are of particular importance with respect to ventilation, aerosol deposition and modifications due to pathological processes.

From inside to outside, the trachea and bronchus are composed of mucosa, lamina propria, submucosa, and tunica fibrocartilaginosa. The mucosa contains mainly cylindrical ciliated epithelial cells which transport mucus and goblet cells which secrete mucus. Under the mucosa, the lamina propria contains a fine network of blood vessels, lymph vessels and nerves with elastic and collagen fibres. The blood and the lymph vessel system are able to absorb aerosol particles. The submucosa contains glandular tissue, especially at points where there is no cartilage. The tracheal cartilages form incomplete rings with smooth muscle that completes their posterior part. Moving distally through the airways, there is a progressive loss of cartilage, mucus-producing elements and cilia. Cartilage disappears at generation 11. The terminal bronchiole is the last fully epithelialized and ciliated airway.

Respiratory bronchioles are covered with ciliated cells and Clara cells constituting a flat epithelium

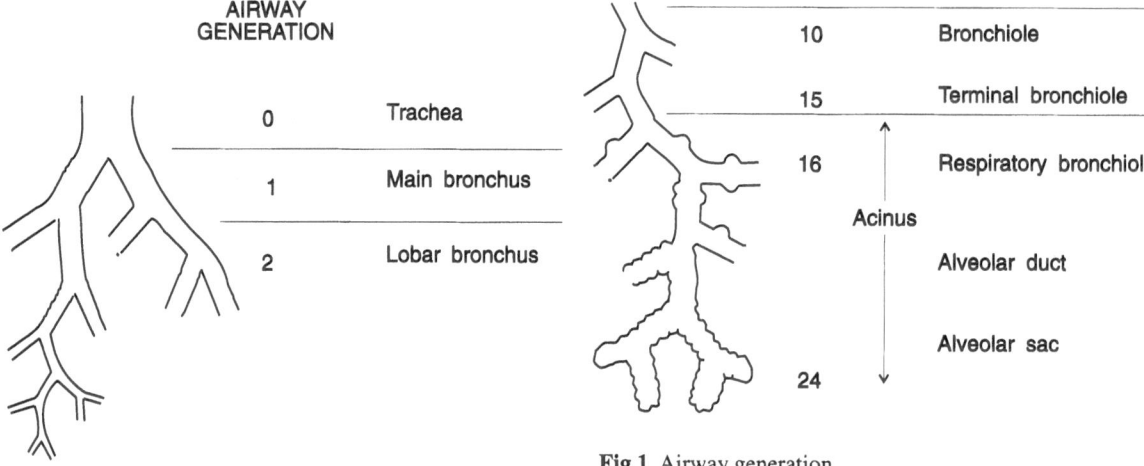

Fig.1. Airway generation

opening into the alveoli. The alveolar epithelium lies on a basement membrane and includes three types of cells. The alveolar epithelial cells (type I) cover the alveolar surface very thinly. The alveolar granulocytes (type II) produce surfactant, a substance that enhances the stability of alveoli and regenerates type I cells. Alveolar macrophages lie on the epithelium surface of the alveoli. The basic unit of the bronchopulmonary structure is termed an acinus. It consists of all airways and lung tissues arising from a single terminal bronchiole. The acinus is the fundamental unit of gas exchange.

Structure and function of the alveolo-capillary region

The alveolocapillary region has an important role not only for gas exchange. The lung is open to the atmosphere air and is also in contact with the circulation. These facts explain pathological data due to external air injury or systemic diseases. The region can be divided into three elements, the alveolar space, the capillaries and the interstitium (fig. 2). The alveolar space is in contact with air and is involved in lung defense mechanisms against inhaled organisms. Alveolar macrophages have a phagocytic function and have an important role in immune defense. This is the case when respiratory injury occurs and also after exposure to inhaled toxic agents (asbestos and beryllium) or inhaled allergens (mouldy hay, mushroom spores, humidifiers, etc). The term alveolitis is commonly used to describe non-infectious diseases with increased cellularity of bronchoalveolar lavage. Tissue damage in alveolitis involves the entire acinus

including the small airways and, in the later stages, fibrosis of the alveolar wall.

At the level of the alveoli, capillaries form a dense network, the basic element of which is a short cylindrical tube, with an internal diameter of 8 μm, lined with endothelial cells. Circulating agents such as cytotoxic agents and drugs are able to provoke alveolitis and fibrosis at a later stage. Their action may be due to direct toxicity or may be immunologically mediated.

The interstitial tissue contains collagen, elastic fibres and a matrix lying between the fibre components. This connective tissue constitutes the framework of the lung and provides adequate tension in the range of breathing volume. When alveolitis and secondary diffuse pulmonary fibrosis occur as a consequence of exposure to toxic agents, allergens or lung involvement of collagen disease, there is hypertrophy of interstitial tissue due to increase in collagen content and migration of cells from blood-macrophages, neutrophils, eosinophils or lymphocytes. Such lung inflammation can be detected by nuclear imaging. Fluid accumulates around the airways and blood vessels in the interstitial space when pulmonary edema occurs.

Lung defense mechanisms

The normal lower respiratory tract is almost always sterile. However, contamination due to bacteria, inhaled organisms, atmospheric pollutants and nasal secretions are common occurrences. Lung defense mechanisms involve the cough reflex, mucociliary

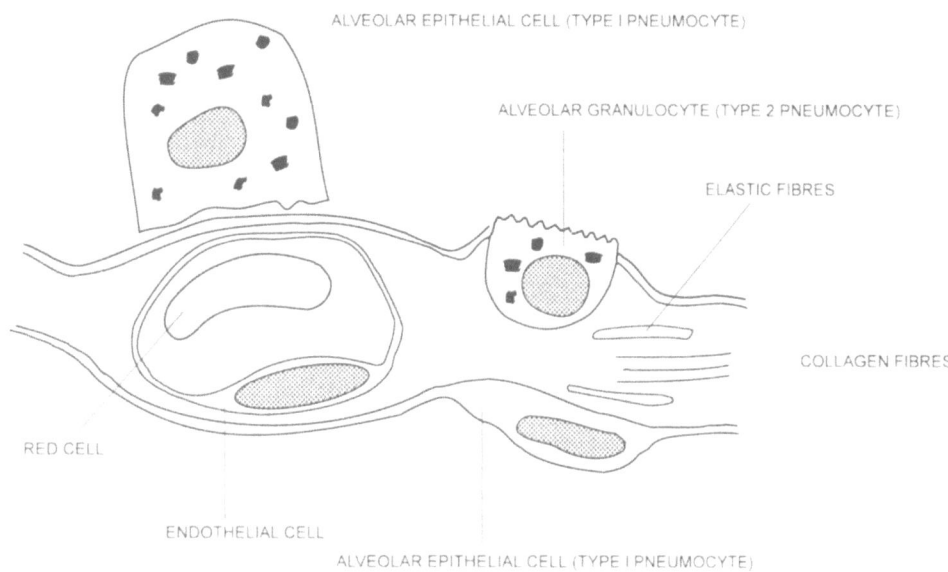

Fig. 2. Structure of the alveolocapillary membrane

clearance in the respiratory tract, phagocytosis and inflammatory reaction in the alveolar compartment.

Mucociliary clearance can clear particles deposited in the tracheobronchial tree very rapidly. It depends on the quantity and quality of mucus produced and the ciliary function. Mucus is a complex material covering the epithelium and propelled forward by cilia beating to eliminate contaminants. It contains antimicrobial proteins, facilitates ciliary action to remove particles and protects the epithelium from injury caused by elements such as irritants or enzymatic degradation. The quality of mucociliary clearance depends on the viscoelastic properties of mucus and ciliary movement. In chronic obstructive pulmonary diseases, both the quantity and viscosity of the secretion increase, impairing normal removal of particles and microorganisms. Impairment of ciliary function occurs with smoking, alcohol, infection and inhaled irritants.

At the alveolar level, inhaled organisms are normally phagocytosed by macrophages with the help of antibacterial factors such as IgG and the complement. In the presence of infection, alveolar macrophages liberate factors which attract other cells such as neutrophils and lymphocytes. Impaired removal of secretions or impaired immune response contribute to the development of infection. In these conditions, normally non-pathogenic organisms may become invasive and pathogenic.

Ventilation

The major role of the respiratory system is to exchange O_2 and CO_2 from the blood passing through the lungs. Gas exchange can be divided into three functional components: ventilation, pulmonary circulation, and the diffusion of O_2 and CO_2 across the alveolar-capillary barrier.

Ventilation consists of the cyclic movement of air from outside through the airways to the alveolar space where gas exchange occurs. The volume of the lung is the sum of two volumes, alveolar volume (AV) and dead space volume (DV). Gas exchange occurs in the alveolar space but not in the dead space which corresponds to the conductive zone of the airways. Under normal conditions and at rest, the dead space ventilation accounts for a third of the total ventilation, two-thirds being used for alveolar ventilation.

The flow of gas coming to and from the alveoli is dependant on the mechanical characterisitics of the lungs and airways and is also dependant on the forces acting on them (muscular forces and inertia of the ventilatory system). The mechanical characterisitics are mainly dependant on the resistance to flow in the airways (R_{AW}) and on the elastic properties of the lung parenchyma. R_{AW} is the quotient of the pressure difference between the mouth (Pm) and the alveoli (Palv) and the associated flow rate ($\dot{V}$): R_{AW} = Pm – Palv/$\dot{V}$. Total airway resistance can be divided into

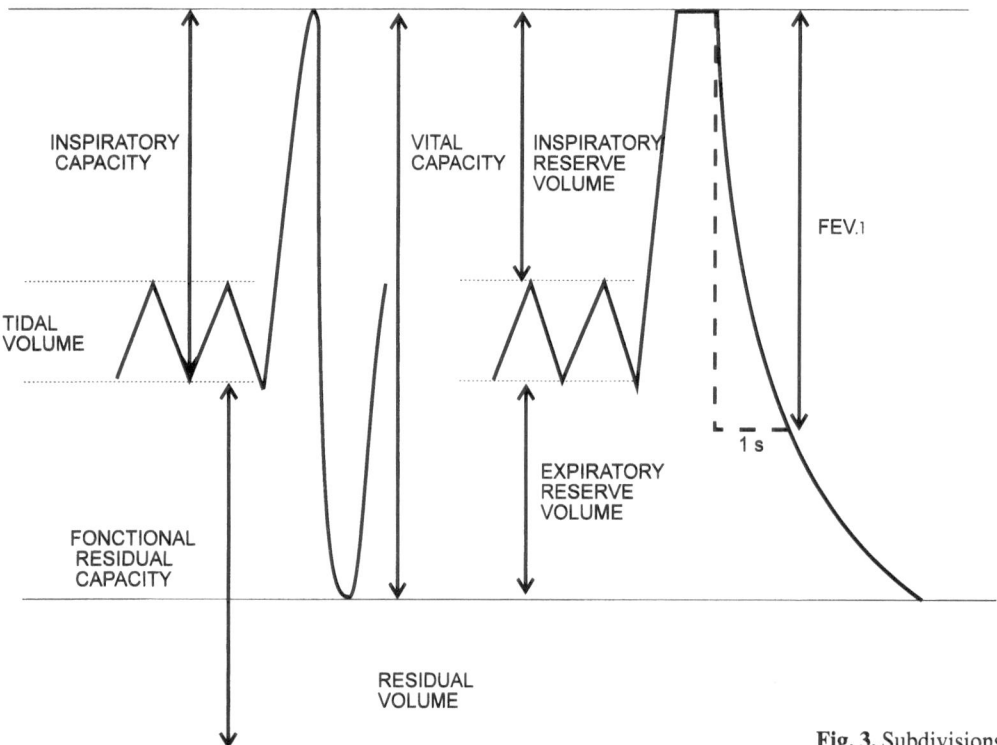

INSPIRATORY
CAPACITY

VITAL
CAPACITY

INSPIRATORY
RESERVE
VOLUME

FEV.1

TIDAL
VOLUME

FONCTIONAL
RESIDUAL
CAPACITY

EXPIRATORY
RESERVE
VOLUME

1 s

RESIDUAL
VOLUME

Fig. 3. Subdivisions of lung volumes

resistance which occurs in the central airways (80 to 90% of total resistance) and resistance due to the laminar flow in the peripheral airways (10 to 20% of total resistance). Airflow obstruction which affects central airways has a marked effect on total resistance.

The elastic properties of the lungs are evaluated by the compliance (C_L). C_L is the quotient of a change in volume and the concomitant change in transpulmonary pressure: $C_L = \Delta V / \Delta P$.

At each lung volume, the transpulmonary pressure is determined from the difference between alveolar air pressure and intra-pleural pressure. Volume-pressure relationships are modified in diseases altering lung tissue elasticity. Emphysema, which is characterized by destruction of the alveolar walls, increases the compliance of the lungs. Conversely, the lungs of patients with pulmonary fibrosis are less distensible.

Lung volumes can be divided into different compartments (fig. 3). During quiet breathing, the volume of air inhaled during inspiration and leaving the lungs during passive expiration, is called tidal volume (V_T). The volume of air remaining in the lung at the end of a spontaneous expiration is termed functional residual capacity (FRC). FRC comprises the expiratory reserve volume (ERV) plus residual volume (RV). RV is the volume of air remaining in the lungs after a maximum expiratory effort. The maximum volume of air which can be inhaled from

midposition is termed the inspiratory capacity (IC). IC comprises V_T plus the inspiratory reserve volume (IRV). The vital capacity (VC) is the maximum volume of air that can be inhaled after a maximum inspiration. The forced expiratory volume in one second (FEV_1) is the volume of air exhaled during the first second of a maximal forced expiration beginning at the end of a complete inspiration. FEV_1, expressed as a percentage of the vital capacity, is an index of expiratory airflow obstruction. V_T, VC, IRV, ERV and FEV_1 can be measured with a simple spirometer giving a spirogram. Data obtained from a spirogram are suitable routinely to evaluate an airflow obstruction. The flow-volume curve is obtained by simultaneously measuring the flow rate in liters per second and lung volumes. The examination of the shape of this curve is very useful. Patients with early lung disease resulting in an airflow obstruction may have normal FEV_1 but the flow-volume curve may be concave. RV and FRC are usually measured by dilution of a non-absorbable tracer gas such as helium in a closed spirometer system during normal quiet breathing. Nevertheless, the best measurements are obtained with a body plethysmograph. The patient is put into an airtight box. Measurements of variation in thorax volume are related to variations in pressure of the intrathoracic gas and of the box.

Disorders of lung ventilation

A restrictive disorder is defined as a decrease in the total lung capacity. It corresponds to a reduction in the number of alveoli (resection) a compression of the lung tissue (pleurisy), and local occlusion of the airways (foreign body). In pulmonary fibrosis, there is a restrictive disorder because the changed elastic properties of the lung tissue result in a limitation of maximum inspiration and maximum expiration.

An obstructive disorder is defined as a decrease in the FEV_1. This abnormality is usually the result of a chronic obstructive pulmonary disease (COPD). The residual volume is usually increased due to inspiratory displacement of the level of breathing at rest. COPD comprise chronic bronchitis and emphysema. Chronic bronchitis is defined as a chronic cough with production of sputum for at least 3 months in the year for at least 2 years.

Anatomic disorder is characterized by hyper-secretion and inflammation of the bronchi caused by irritants, mainly by cigarette exposure. Emphysema is a pathological diagnosis. Two types of emphysema are described according to the location of the disease. In centrolobular emphysema, the damage primarily affects the respiratory bronchioles. The consequence is disturbance of ventilation-perfusion relationships and hypoxia. In panlobular emphysema, there is destruction of the entire acinus. This destruction is related to the balance of enzyme systems in the lung in which a deficiency of $\alpha 1$-antitrypsin, an antielastase, has a predominant role.

Circulation

Pulmonary circulation is closely related to ventilation structure in order to allow gas exchange. The pulmonary blood pressure is about one-sixth of that in the systemic circulation due to a low resistance to flow. The pulmonary blood vessels are highly elastic and larger than the systemic vessels and the vascular bed has a very high perfusion capacity. This low-pressure system is heavily dependant on physiopathologic factors such as gravitation, physical exertion, hypoxia, acidosis and drug effects. Blood flow is greater in the base than in the apex of the upright lung. During physical exertion in a young man, an increase in the pulmonary blood flow rate from 6 l/min at rest to about 40 l/min causes no rise in the pulmonary artery pressure because of the remarkable capacity of the pulmonary capillaries to dilate. In contrast, hypoxia causes a rise in the resistance to flow and thus an increase in the pulmonary pressure. Administration of drugs such as adrenalin and α-sympathicomimetics are able to increase the pulmonary blood pressure whereas acetylcholine dilates constricted arterioles. In response to environmental factors, the resistance of the pulmonary circulation can be modified by the distension or recruitment of pulmonary vessels previously closed or by closure of vessels previously open.

Regional distribution of pulmonary blood flow can be measured by injecting radiolabeled particles which are just too large to pass through the pulmonary arteries. They are retained in proportion to the blood flow. Thus the external count of the lungs reflects the regional flow. An alternative method is the injection of ^{133}Xe, which leaves the body by diffusion through the alveolar-capillary barrier, and therefore the regional lung activity reflects the regional blood flow.

Gas diffusion

Alveolar-capillary diffusion is a process in which gas molecules move across the air space to the capillaries and vice versa. The alveolar wall is normally 0.1 to 0.5 μm thick. The transport of gas through the alveolar-capillary membrane is determined by the following factors: alveolar-capillary gas pressure gradient, solubility and molecular weight of the gas and thickness and composition of the alveolar-capillary membrane. This membrane represents a resistance to diffusion.

The partial pressure of carbon dioxide is 5.3 kPa (40 mm Hg) in arterial blood and 6.1 kPa (45 mm Hg) in venous blood. The carbonic acid dissociation curve shows a linear relationship between CO_2 content and CO_2 pressure in the physiological range. The high solubility of CO_2 gives a rate of diffusion about 20 times that of oxygen. Thus the membrane factor plays a limited role in the alveolar-capillary transport of CO_2. In contrast, CO_2 exchange is limited by the chemical binding to hemoglobin in blood and the capillary blood flow.

Alveolar-capillary oxygen transport is limited by the low rate of diffusion through the alveolar-capillary membrane, its combination with hemoglobin in blood and the capillary blood flow. Oxygen transport is very sensitive to disturbances in lung function, as a result of its transfer properties. In lung diseases such as fibrosis, sarcoidosis and interstitial edema, the alveolar-capillary barrier appears under the microscope to be thickened. The alveolar-capillary transport of oxygen is disturbed, involving an abnormally large oxygen gradient between the alveoli and the end-capillary blood. In contrast, CO_2 diffusion is disturbed only in severe pathological conditions, due to its high solubility. In fact, membrane thickening alone is not sufficient to explain the impairment of oxygen diffusion if there are no ventilation-perfusion disturbances. Arterial hypoxemia in these patients is essentially due to abnormalities of ventilation-perfusion ratio.

Diffusing capacity can be estimated using the measurement of carbon monoxide diffusion. It is reduced by thickening or edema of the alveolar-capillary membrane and by emphysematous lesions which increase the distance for gas diffusion and decrease the alveolar-capillary area.

Ventilation – perfusion relationships

Maximal efficiency of gas exchange occurs when both ventilation and perfusion are equally distributed in all regions of the lungs. Even in normal patients this is not the case because there are differences in ventilation and perfusion between the bottom and the top due to the effects of gravity in the upright posture. In alveoli at the top of the lung, alveolar ventilation is about three times greater than blood flow. In these conditions O_2 uptake by capillary blood and a CO_2 output are relatively higher because of higher ventilation. This phenomenon is reversed at the bottom of the lung where alveolar ventilation is less than capillary blood flow O_2 uptake. In fact, in normal lung patients, these variations in ventilation-perfusion ratios are small and do not really influence PO_2. On the other hand, in lung diseases, decreases in PO_2 are often due to alteration of ventilation-perfusion ratio.

In normal subjects, the ratio of alveolar ventilation in liters per minute to pulmonary blood flow in liters per minute (AV/Q) is about 0.8. This ratio normally varies from 0.5 in the lung base to 3.0 in the lung apex. Theoretically, under pathological conditions, all possible ventilation-perfusion ratios can be shown from zero (shunt circulation) to infinity (dead space ventilation). In clinical investigation, the ventilation-perfusion ratios are divided into three categories:

– $A\dot{V}/\dot{Q}$ is normal at rest. During physical exertion, ventilation and perfusion increase equally;

– $A\dot{V}/\dot{Q}$ is decreased (shunt circulation) as the result of patchy abnormalities in airway resistance or lung compliance which reduces ventilation. O_2 uptake

and CO_2 output are reduced. Perfusion is normal and sometimes increased indicating compensatory hyperfunction;

– $A\dot{V}/\dot{Q}$ is increased (dead space ventilation) as a result of obstruction (embolism) or obliteration of pulmonary blood vessels, which reduce pulmonary blood flow. The alveoli are normally ventilated but not perfused.

Assessment of regional ventilation and perfusion can be performed by gas analysis and gaseous radio-nuclide methods. Due to the high diffusion capacity of CO_2, inequalities of ventilation perfusion in the lungs cause a low PaO_2, but Pa CO_2 may be normal, even lower than normal if arterial hypoxia stimulates breathing. $PaCO_2$ can be used to define the level of alveolar ventilation. An increase in $PaCO_2$ value reveals hypoventilation whereas hyperventilation is defined as a decrease in $PaCO_2$ below normal values.

Radiolabeled gas, introduced into the lungs via the ventilation or the circulation, emits gamma rays which can be measured outside the thorax and are suitable for the study of the regional function of the lungs. It is of great value because gas with different characteristics can be labeled for specific purposes. The relative volumes, ventilation and circulation are measured in terms of space and time.

Aerosols

Ventilation can be imaged in vivo by isotopic methods based on inhalation of radio-active aerosols or gases.

An aerosol is a physical system of solid particles or liquid droplets with a small enough diameter to remain in suspension in the atmosphere.

Aerosol properties

Aerosols can theoretically be characterized by single or collective particle properties. The chemical or, possibly more interesting in terms of aerosol kinetics, physical properties of single particles can be analyzed. Liquid particles are sphere shaped and their size is simply characterized by radius, diameter, surface and volume.

Their terminal settling velocity is an important physical characteristic. It depends upon gravitational and viscous forces and is easy to calculate taking into account these two well-defined parameters. Solid particles can also be spherical or of more complicated shape. Spheroidal solid particles are describable by two parameters. Some solid particles have such a

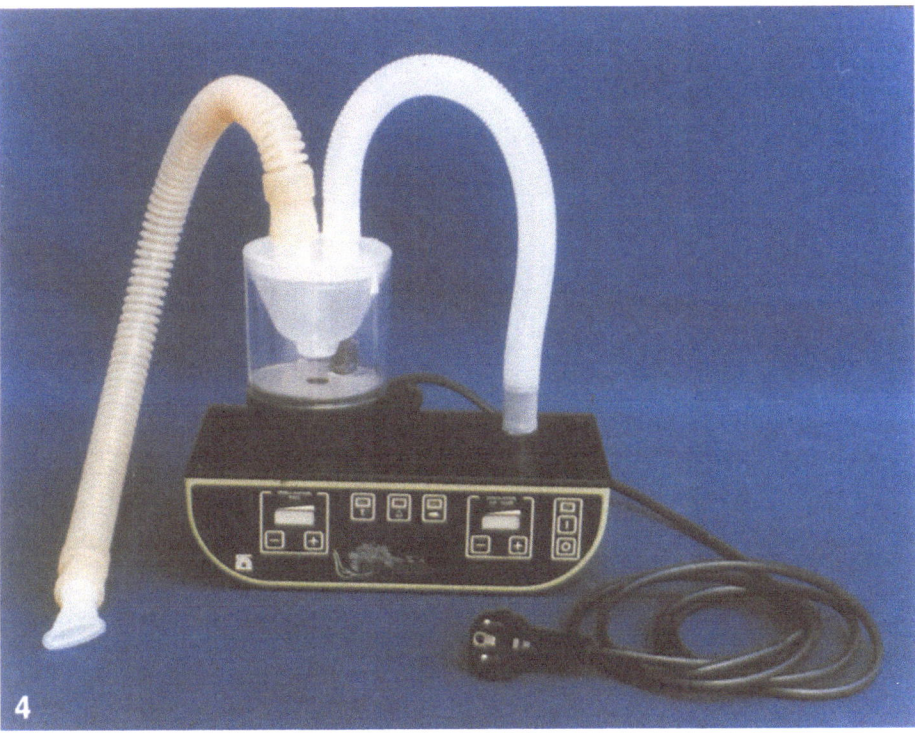

Fig. 4. DP100® (DP Medical, France) ultrasonic nebuliser operating at 2.4 MHz frequency

complex shape that size is difficult to evaluate mathematically. One method in this case is to relate inertia behaviour of the particle to a sphere. This is the concept of aerodynamic equivalent diameter (AED). AED is the diameter of a sphere of unit density ($1g/cm^3$) which has the same settling velocity in the same gas. Particles of equal AED are dynamically identical. Other individual properties such as electric charge and Brownian motion are important in terms of aerosol kinetics.

By statistical analysis, collective properties of aerosols corresponding to a great number of particles can be characterized. Several criteria can be used. The number concentration is the number of particles per cubic centimeter. Usually particles are separated by a distance at least 10 times the diameter of particles and there are 10^4 - 10^7 particles per cubic centimeter. The mass concentration is expressed as the mass of aerosol per cubic meter of air. Size distribution is represented as a histogram with the size-range on the horizontal axis and the number or percentage of particles on the vertical axis. Size-range is chosen according to the size resolution and generally distributed in a geometric progression as the majority of aerosols are geo-metrically rather than arithmetically distributed. When nearly all particles fall into one range, the aerosol is monodisperse. This is rare with medical aerosols. Most medical aerosols are heteropolydisperse. The size distribution is more often not symmetrical but skewed, with a long tail for larger sizes and dropping to zero for smaller sizes. This is due to the fact that distribution is log normal, meaning that distribution is the logarithm of particle size. Nevertheless, mathematical concepts can be employed to describe aerosols more precisely in terms of size. Some, such as median size, mode size and standard deviation, are very usual. Count median size (CMD) separates distribution into two halves, the one with a lower size and the other with a larger size. As distribution is log normal, geometric standard deviation (Sg) replaces the usual standard deviation in arithmetic normal distribution. Some criteria more specific to the aerosol field have been defined. Median size for mass (MMAD) is widely used. It divides the actual mass of aerosol into two halves. This parameter is very useful to define therapeutic aerosols, the effects of which are dose dependant.

CMD or MMAD and properties related to them can be evaluated by several methods. Electron microscopy is used for the measurement of spherical particles. Two

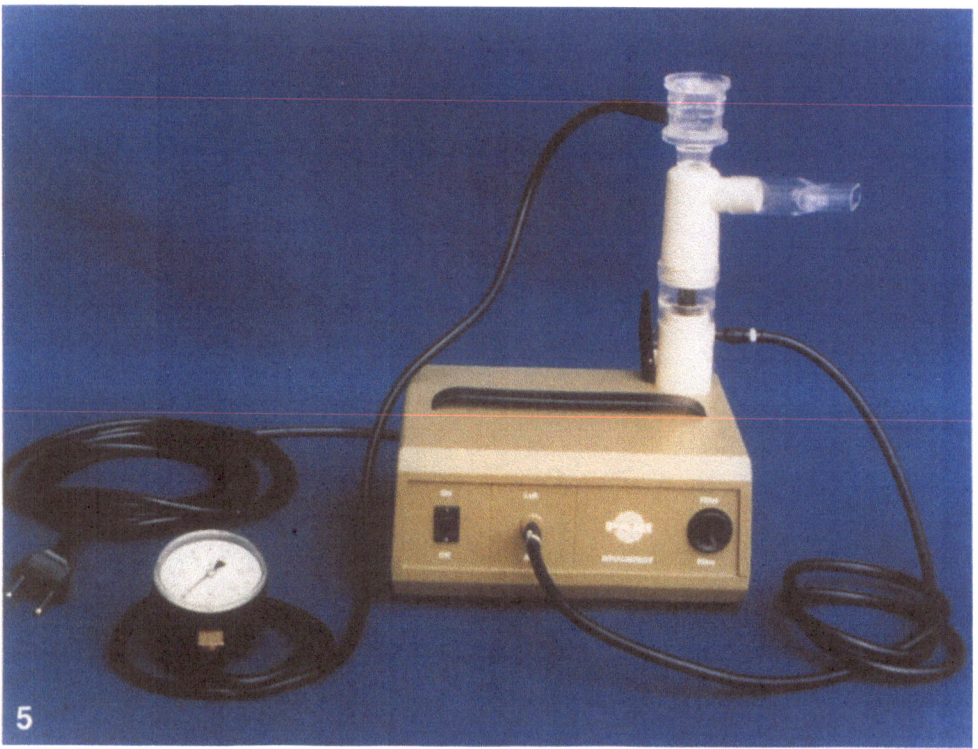

Fig. 5. Pari boy® (Pari, Germany) jet nebuliser

other methods, laser light-scattering particle sizers and cascade impactors, are available whatever the shape of particles. Due to technical specificities, results obtained by these 2 techniques do not always fit and there is still some controversy concerning the definition of the standard.

Aerosol generators

Medical aerosol generators are based on a comminution process which results from the break-up of a solid or, more often, liquid phase.

For therapeutic use, commercial systems such as metered dose inhalers or, more recently, dry powdered inhalers (spinhaler, diskhaler, rotahaler, turbuhaler, etc) are available. These systems, prepared for use with a pharmacologically active substances, are not usable as a diagnostic tool.

Jet nebulizers and ultrasonic nebulizers are usable for pulmonary nuclear medicine. With both these systems, the solution for aerosolization is put into a chamber the volume of which ranges from 5 ml to 700 ml.

With pneumatic (jet) nebulizers (fig. 5), aero-solization results from the Bernouilli effect induced by a high velocity air jet. MMAD is inversely proportional to the air flow, which ranges from 5 l/mn to 10 l/mn. When equipped with baffles which remove larger particles, jet nebulizers can produce log-normal distributed aerosols with 1 μm MMAD. Most medical aerosols are aqueous. Therefore, they are cooled with a pressured air jet to a temperature of 15°C below ambient conditions

With ultrasonic nebulizers (fig. 4), aerosolization results from atomization of the solution under the effect of an oscillating piezoelectric crystal. The solution to be aerosolized is put into a thin plastic sheet and coupled to the crystal through water. The MMAD is inversely proportional to the oscillating frequency of the quartz. For peripheral deposition, a frequency of at least 1 Mhz is required.

Mechanisms of aerosol deposition

Particles of 10 μm and above are trapped by impaction in the nose and nasopharynx. Particles of 2 to 10 μm deposit by impaction and sedimentation in the intrathoracic airways. Particles of 0.2 to 5 μm deposit by a sedimentation process after the fourth generation bronchi. Only particles smaller than 2 μm can reach the lung. Particles smaller than 0.1 μm are submitted to Brownian movements in the alveolar compartment.

In conclusion aerosol devices used in nuclear medicine have to be chosen according to the objective of the study. Alveolar-capillary clearance studies for example require very small particles whereas muco ciliary clearance requires larger particles that deposit centrally.

Principles of the imaging process and analysis of images

S Bardet, F Baulieu, N Caillat-Vigneron, S Coequyt, P Diot, JJ Lafitte and P Peltier

Lung scintigraphy gives the clinician valuable tools in the diagnosis or management of major pulmonary disorders. The imaging test agents used allow the imaging of pulmonary perfusion and ventilation.

Perfusion scintigraphy [1]

Perfusion lung scanning was developed by Taplin in 1964 [2]. Small particulate aggregates of albumin or microsphere labeled with technetium-99m were found to be satisfactory test agents for lung perfusion imaging in man.

The size of the particles is critical to the success of studies: macroaggregates - average diameter = 45 μm (large range of size), microspheres - average diameter = 15 μm(small range of sizes). Arterial branching terminates in precapillaries that flow into a network of capillaries. The average diameter of precapillaries and capillaries is respectively 10 μm and 5 μm. After intravenous injection, the particles pass through the right heart and into the lung. Because of their size, 90% of the particles are trapped in the pulmonary precapillary bed [3]. Given that there are about 300 million precapillaries, with a usual dose approximately 1 in 10,000 precapillaries is micro-embolized by the injected particles, an insignificant hemodynamic load.

The distribution of activity reflects the perfusion during the first lung pass and consequently depends on the position of the patient. It is affected by gravity. When the patient is in a supine position, blood pressures become equal in the apical and basal lung regions, and the distribution of pulmonary blood flow becomes uniform in healthy subjects. Conversely, in a sitting position, perfusion may predominate in the bases. To avoid such artefacts, the tracer should be injected in the supine position. The particles must be evenly distributed in the syringe, and blood should not be drawn back into the syringe. If small blood clots are injected with this labeled material, small areas of microembolization may be visualized. Imaging should be performed rapidly after injection. The half-life of reticuloendothelial clearance of particles too small to be trapped in the lung is short and the background counts from the circulating tracer are rapidly non-significant. Macroaggregates are biodegradable. Their pulmonary biological half-life normally ranges between 4 and 8 hrs [3].

Technetium-99m albumin macroaggregates are widely accepted as the perfusion tracer of choice. The usual injected dose is 111 MBq (3mCi); six and/or eight views for perfusion studies have been shown to provide an accurate diagnosis. In addition to the anterior, posterior and lateral views, the posterior and anterior oblique studies have been found to contribute to the definition of perfusion abnormalities [4]; 400 K counts per anterior and posterior image, and 350 K counts per lateral and oblique image have provided sufficient detail for detection of perfusion abnormalities.

In supine control subjects, the distribution of activity is nearly even side to side and apex to base (fig. 1). In patients, abnormalities of perfusion, i.e. hypoperfusioned areas, are detected. Scintigraphy is a sensitive but non-specific method for detecting abnormalities of pulmonary perfusion. Localized defects are seen in regions of pulmonary embolism

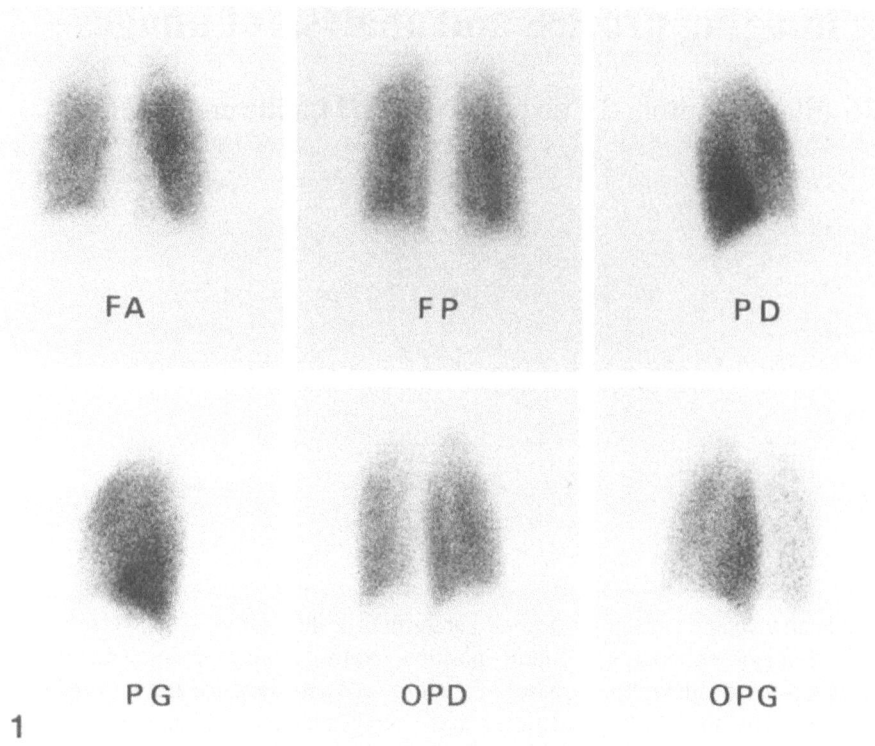

Fig. 1. Normal six-view perfusion lung scan. *FA* anterior, *PD* right lateral, *OPD* right posterior oblique, *FP* posterior, *PG* left lateral, *OPG* left posterior oblique

(figs. 2, 3). They also are seen in regions of parenchymal lung consolidation or collapse, and in other disorders such as reflex vasocontriction secondary to local alveolar hypoxia.

Ventilation scintigraphy [1]

Pulmonary ventilation imaging was introduced by Denardo et al in 1970 [5]. The overall diagnostic accuracy of pulmonary scintigraphic studies is improved when ventilation studies are added to the perfusion imaging. However, in comparison with perfusion scintigraphy, ventilation imaging is less widely used; its procedure is far more complex and more controversial, its protocol lacks standardization and it may be performed after the inhalation of radioactive gas or microparticles.

Radioactive gases

Xenon-133

The most often used radioactive gas is xenon-133. It is relatively inexpensive; its long half-life (5.27 days) permits storage for emergency studies.

One disadvantage is its low photon energy (81 Kev), resulting in reduced scintigraphic resolution. Moreover, because this energy is below that of ^{99m}Tc, it has to be used before perfusion scan.

Imaging is usually performed from the posterior view. Several techniques of xenon administration may be used [6]. The main procedures consist of the single breath technique and the equilibration time method.

Single breath technique

The patient is instructed to take a single breath of the radioactive gas (500 to 1200 MBq) and hold his breath for 10 to 20 sec. During inspiration, the radioactive gas enters various regions of the lung, at a rate directly related to ventilation. This technique is limited only to cooperative patients.

Equilibration time method

The patient inhales the xenon gas (200 MBq/l), from a closed system xenon rebreathing apparatus.

He rebreathes the xenon until a constant lung concentration has been achieved. This is the wash-in phase. At equilibrium, all lung segments have the same tracer concentration and the activity becomes independant of ventilation; the distribution of the

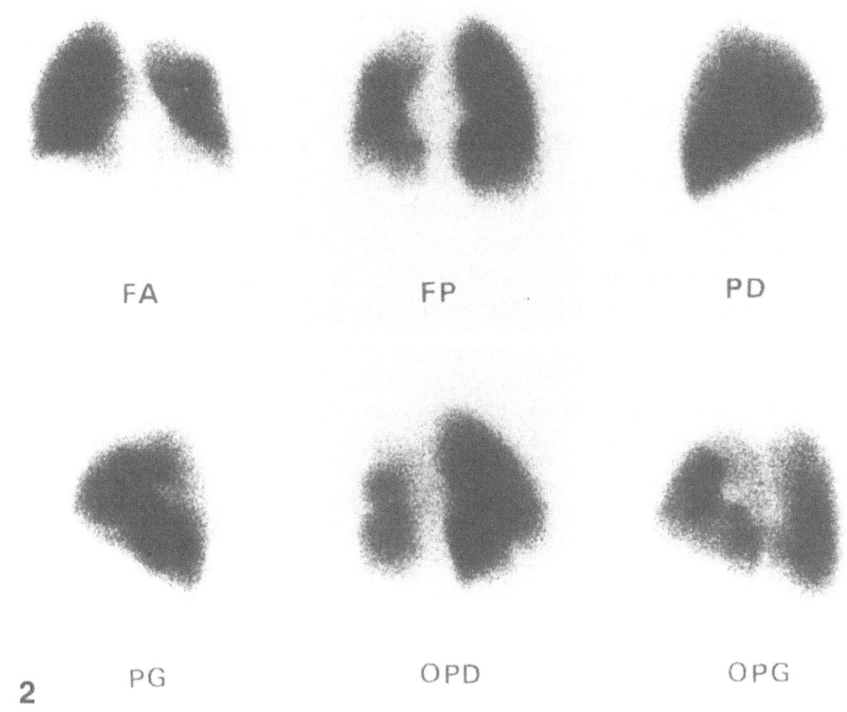

Fig. 2. Perfusion scan in a patient with pulmonary embolism: it reveals a left upper lobe defect. The lobar perfusion defect is clearly seen in anterior, posterior, and oblique posterior views. *FA* anterior, *PD* right lateral, *OPD* right posterior oblique, *FP* posterior, *PG* left lateral, *OPG* left posterior oblique

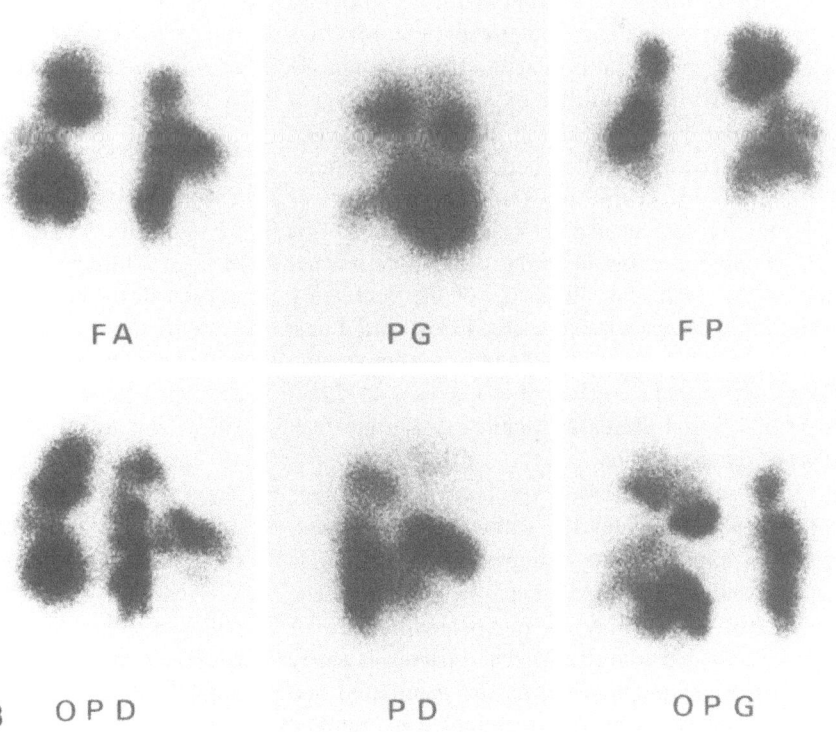

Fig. 3. Six-view perfusion scan in a patient with pulmonary embolism: multiple and segmental defects can be seen in all views. *FA* anterior, *PD* right lateral, *OPD* right posterior oblique, *FP* posterior, *PG* left lateral, *OPG* left posterior oblique

tracer gives an indication of the regional volume of the lung. In controls, a two minute wash-in is normally enough to obtain the equilibrium phase. Finally, after 3 or 4 minutes, the system is opened, and the patient breathes room air normally; the xenon is washed out of the lung. During the wash-out phase, the rate of loss of xenon is proportional to regional ventilation. The wash-out images are indicators of the dead air spaces of the lung. Wash-out imaging has been shown to be a sensitive indicator of ventilatory dysfunction. The difference between the well and poorly ventilated lung segments is obvious only in the inhalation and wash-out phase.

Computer processing methods are necessary to measure regional ventilation and to assess regional clearance times [7, 8].

Because xenon-133 has a long half-life and a ß emission, it requires special equipment for radio-protection.

Krypton-81m

Krypton-81m is a gas with a very short half-life (13 sec), and a γ emission (190 Kev) that results in a good scintigraphic resolution, comparable with that of ^{99m}Tc (140 Kev). It can be used post-perfusion [9].

A cooperative patient is not required. The study is performed as follows: a nose-mouth mask is placed over the patient's face and the patient breathes normally. Krypton-81m is eluted from a rubidium-81 generator, with humidified oxygen. The oxygen/krypton mixture is merged with the existing oxygen supply. Because of the ultra short half-life of krypton-81m, an equilibrium between alveolar tracer concentration and inhaled air is never obtained. This gas can only reflect instantaneous ventilation. It is not suitable for evaluating all phases of the ventilatory cycle. Thus, compared with xenon-133, it would be a less sensitive test in the detection of obstructive lung disease. As a matter of fact, it is less easy to detect areas of krypton decreased ventilatory activity than areas of xenon retention.

Krypton-81m offers several advantages over xenon-133. It provides the patient with minimum radiation exposure; no radioprotection system is required and patient cooperation is not necessary. The ventilation study may be performed before or following the perfusion study. The imaging is easily obtained under multiple views; the ventilation and perfusion images may be superimposed in multiple projections [10].

Conversely, this tracer has a huge disavantage. It is produced from a rubidium-81 generator which is expensive and has a half-life of only 4.7 hr. It must be supplied daily, its availability is limited to the centers in the vicinity of cyclotrons. Finally it is very expensive, and has a limited availability, making it impractical for emergency use.

Labeled aerosols

The concept of labeled aerosols is not at all a new concept [3]. However, their satisfactory use is relatively recent. For a long time the problem was the ability to produce submicron particles. An aerosol is a suspension of solid particles. The distribution of the aerosol through the respiratory tract depends on the size of the particles. Particles larger than 10 μm are trapped in the nasopharynx; particles ranging in size from 5 and 10 μm are retained in the trachea and bronchi; the small particles, with a caliber smaller than 2 μm, are retained in the alveoli. For ventilation lung imaging, the radioactive aerosol is mainly composed of particles ranging in size from 0.1 to 2 μm. Technetium labeled aerosols can be administered either before or after perfusion scanning. However the amount of activity that is placed in the nebulizer is much greater when the ventilation is performed after perfusion imaging. Technetium-99m DTPA aerosols (Venticis™) have become quite popular for ventilation imaging. Another preparation, technetium-99m carbon particles (Technegas™) may be used for ventilation imaging.

Radioaerosol of technetium-99 m Venticis™ [11]

The radioactive agent, DTPA or colloidal sulphur, labeled with ^{99m}Tc, is introduced into a nebulizer through a filling tube. The nebulizer is aerated at an oxygen flow-rate of 8-10 l/min; with the Venticis™ system, the submicronic aerosol is composed of particles with a median diameter of 0.80 μm and a geometric standard deviation of 2.1. In a pre-perfusion study, the nebulizer should be filled with about 10^3 MBq (30 mCi). In a post-perfusion study, a much larger amount of activity up to 3 x 10^3 MBq (75 mCi), must be placed in the nebulizer. Imaging is easily performed in multiple projections.

However radioaerosols are not gases. Their pulmonary deposition is influenced by the mass of particles and by the patterns of regional ventilation. In normal subjects, pulmonary activity is homogeneous and the lung images after radioaerosol inhalation and macroaggregate perfusion are nearly identical. In patients with obstructive broncho-pulmonary disease, the turbulent air flow in large airways can induce excessive local deposition. On the other hand, another disadvantage is the absence of wash-out images.

Radioaerosol scintigraphy has several advantages; the radioaerosol system is simple, compact and relatively inexpensive. The particles are labeled with 99mTc.

In addition to these desired physical characterisitics, radioaerosol scintigraphy has some disadvantages; the system is relatively inefficient and a large amount of technetium has to be administered, specially after a perfusion study. In the case of broncho-pulmonary disease, aerosol is not the ideal indicator of regional ventilatory performance, because of the possibility of central significant activity deposition.

Technegas™ [12]

Radioaerosols are impaired by some limitations, namely particle size and the specific radioactivity within the carrier gas.

Techegas uses technetium-99m eluate in a graphite crucible and produces a structured ultrafine dispersion with a very small particle size (about 5 nm). On inhalation, the particles adhere to the alveolar walls and therefore multiple conventional views can be performed. In comparison with DTPA aerosols, the count statistics are improved. It would be a good agent for the study of inhalation dynamics and would offer an advance in the investigation of pulmonary disorders.

However, the Technegas system is expensive, which may reduce its practical use.

Gallium scintigraphy

Technical considerations

Gallium-67 is a metal that resembles the ferric ion in atomic radius and charge. As the ferric ion can easily be reduced in vivo, gallium remains bound to iron transport proteins and carrier molecules: transferrin, lactoferrin, ferritin and siderophores [13]. In 1969 Edwards and Hayes first described thoracic localization of gallium-67 in Hodgkin's disease [14] and since then gallium-67 scanning has been widely used for the imaging of neoplasms and the diagnosis of inflammatory disease. Nevertheless, the mechanism facilitating the transfer from plasma to malignant cells or inflammatory lesions still remains controversial.

Gallium-67, usually injected as a citrate to faci-

litate solubilization, has a physical half-life of seventy-eight hours and is a pure gamma emitter. The probability of emitting a photon is less than one per disintegration and simultaneous detection of the three main photopeaks (93, 184 and 296 KeV) greatly improve the statistical content of the image. This is best achieved by using three separate 20% pulse-height analyzer windows.

The amount of activity used for detection of suspected inflammatory or tumoral lesions varies from 74 to 370 MBq according to authors and the method of detection. Imaging is best performed forty-eight hours to seventy-two hours after intravenous administration with a multipeak large field Anger camera equipped with a suitable medium energy collimator. Ten to twenty-five percent of the injected dose is excreted in the urine within the first twenty-four hours, with slower subsequent excretion primarily via the bowel. Large bowel clearance by use of oral laxatives is indicated starting on the day of injection of the radionuclide and continuing until imaging is completed.

Conventional multiple anterior, posterior and oblique camera views performed at least forty-eight hours after intra-venous injection on a well-prepared patient provide most of the information. Delayed imaging after administration of enemas or tomographic projections can be performed when information is not easily obtained or localized from routine examination. The tomographic procedure needs a specific large dose to be injected and does not ever improve the quality of the information of the gallium scan.

Normal gallium-67 regional imaging

Forty-eight to seventy-two hours after intravenous injection, the uptake of gallium-67 in the lung is normally low, indistinguishable from the background activity. Most of the radionuclide retained in the body is distributed within the bone marrow of the entire skeleton and in the liver [15, 16] (fig. 4).

Lateral or oblique views may help to distinguish normal uptake by the sternum from mediastinal lesions, especially in cases of inflammatory anemia with enhancement of bone-marrow uptake of the gallium ion bound to transferrin.

The liver uptake of gallium depends on the catabolism of transferrin and lactoferrin. Usually reliable and homogeneous, it can vary from one patient's clinical status to another and does not need to be kept as a reference for quantification of regional

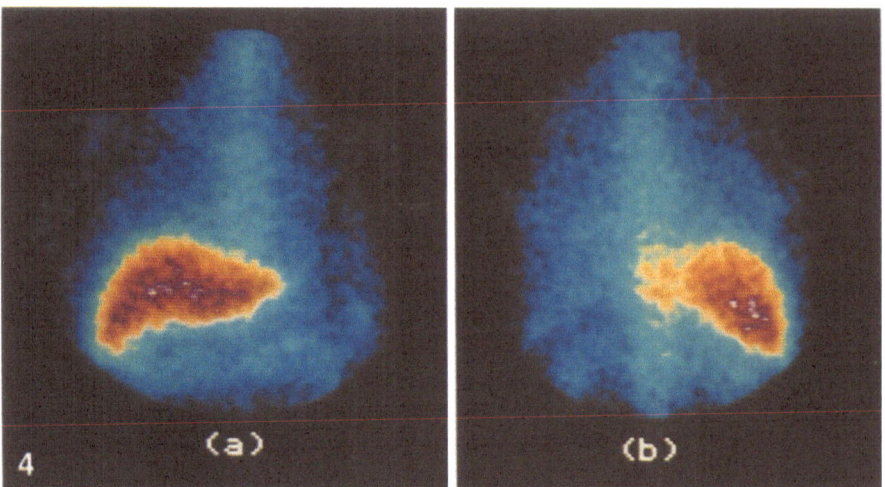

Fig. 4. Normal Gallium-67 thoracic imaging. Anterior view *(a)* and posterior view *(b):* no pathological lung or mediastinal uptake. Gallium-67 activity is distributed within the bone marrow (rib cage, spine and scapulae) and the liver

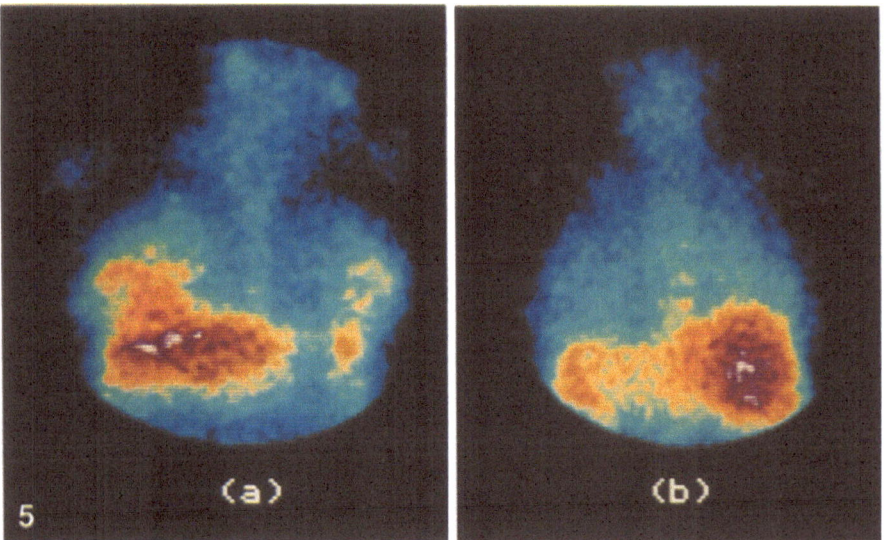

Fig. 5. Gallium-67 thoracic imaging, normal variant. Anterior view *(a)* and posterior view *(b):* prominent uptake of Gallium-67 in breast tissue without any abnormality

gallium-67 uptake. The normal spleen does not retain gallium but a slight uptake may be observed after chemotherapy or under any other circumstance stimulating the reticuloendothelial system.

Oily contrast medium used in lymphography might provide a prominent lung uptake and a false positive gallium-scan related to local vascular reactions.

Faint to intense localization of gallium-67 in the breast tissue of many women may occur without any breast abnormality and should be considered as a normal variant (fig. 5). The intensity of this uptake

seems to be particularly dependent on the menarche or the administration of estro-progestational drugs and could be related to the binding of the gallium ion to lactoferrin.

In children, gallium-67 is distributed in normal thymic tissue. The pattern of this uptake is variable and could be confusing in the exploration of a mediastinal mass seen on chest X-ray. As gallium concentrates in actively dividing young cells in relation to the number of membrane transferrin receptors, the uptake in the growth plates near the epiphyseal regions of long

Table 1. Estimates of absorbed radiation doses (in mGy per 37 MBq intravenous injection of gallium-67). After Summerville D A and Treves S T (1988) in pediatric applications with a minimum dose of 9.25 MBq and a maximum dose of 111MBq [5]. After MIRD dose estimate report number 2 (1973) for adult applications, (experimental results established for homogeneous distribution of the tracer within the body organs) [6].

Age (years)	Newborn	1	5	10	Adult
Body weight (kg)	3.5	9.4	19	32	70
Small intestine	24	19	10	6.7	3.6
Large intestine	120	55.3	29	17	5.6
Kidneys	44	24	14.5	9.2	4.1
Liver	52	29	15.8	10.8	4.6
Red marrow	–	57.9	28.9	16.9	5.8
Spleen	84	36.8	21	13.1	5.3
Ovaries	25.2	16	8.7	5.8	2.8
Testes	20	11	5.6	3.6	2.4
Total body	28	3.9	7.8	4.9	2.6

bones is prominent. The absorbed dose from intravenous injection of gallium-67 in the red marrow, the bone surface and the growing plates has to be kept in mind when discussing the benefit of a gallium scan in a child.

Toxicity and dosimetry of gallium-67

Neither toxicity nor adverse effects have been reported after intravenous injection of gallium-67 when using nuclear medicine doses. The question of radiation load has been much disputed in the past. At present the fields of clinical interest for gallium-67 imaging have been established and the indications for application have to be selected very carefully, especially regarding children.The biological distribution, uptake and retention of radiopharmaceuticals vary considerably throughout childhood, particularly with gallium-67, and dosimetric considerations may modify the risk-benefit ratio for a child (table 1).

Thoracic imaging with gallium-67

First used for the imaging of a variety of epithelial and lymphoreticular neoplasms, gallium-67 localizes in inflammatory lesions as well. The uptake of this radionuclide is not restricted by anatomical barriers and interference with transferrin receptors on the cell membranes is suggested as the primary reason for its accumulation [17]. Increased capillary permeability and direct bacterial uptake may be other contributing factors.

However, gallium-67 imaging of the thorax is used for a number of indications:

To assess hilar and mediastinal involvement in pulmonary malignancies

There is little clinical value in investigating gallium-67 uptake in primary lung cancer, as high resolution computerized tomography detects smaller lesions. The pattern of gallium distribution is altered by radiation therapy and cytotoxic drugs. Hepatic activity can obscure lesions in the right lower lobe and there is no uptake in necrotic lesions. Gallium-67 is less sensitive than chest radiographs in detecting pulmonary dissemination of tumors and mediastinal staging should only be used in selected cases.

To assess extent and to follow up progression or response in the course of a lymphomatous disease

Gallium imaging is at least as sensitive or even more sensitive than radiography in detecting mediastinal and pulmonary involvement of Hodgkin's disease and non-Hodgkin's lymphomas. The variation of uptake in lesions may be related to the grade of malignancy of the lymphoma [18] but some cell receptors could play a major role [19]. A positive gallium scintigraphy after therapy may be the only objective evidence of persistence or recurrence of the disease. Late post-irradiation fibrosis can be distinguished from a recurrent tumor since the former is gallium-negative and the latter is usually Gallium-positive [20].

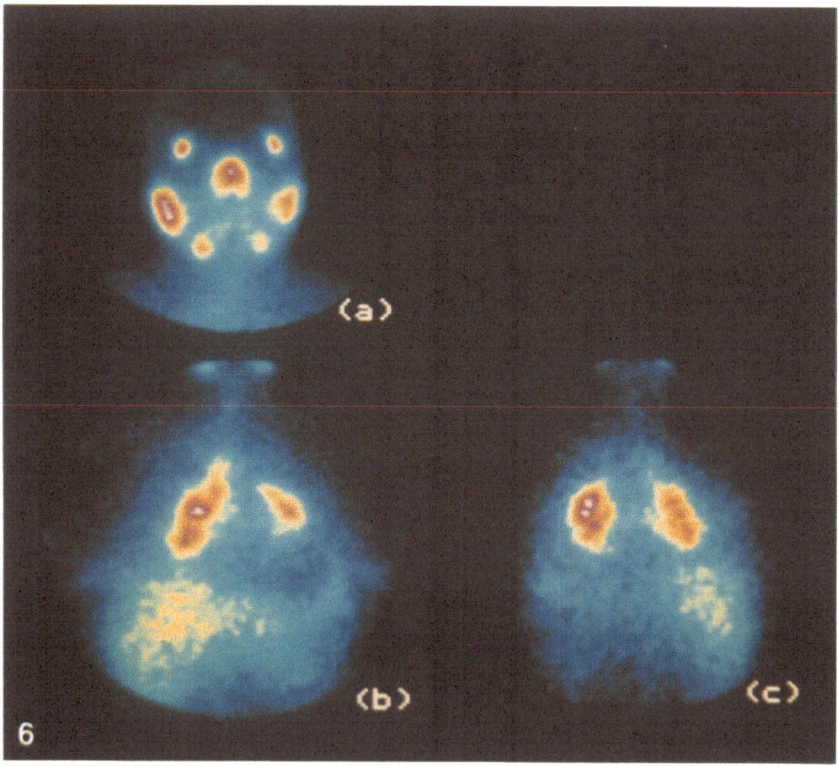

Fig. 6. Gallium-67 uptake in sarcoïdosis. Anterior view of the head *(a)*: Gallium-67 uptake of lacrymal and salivary glands (panda pattern). Anterior view *(b)* and posterior view *(c)* of the chest : right paratracheal (azygous) and para- and infrahilar (intrapulmonary) lymphnode uptake (lambda pattern)

To assess extent, location and inflammatory activity of diffuse interstitial lung disease of various origins

First, sarcoidosis is strongly suggested by the typical combination of pulmonary and salivary gland uptake often recognized as simultaneous "panda" and "lambda" gallium-67 uptake image (fig. 6). Furthermore, in therapy follow-up, relapse can be diagnosed or, when uptake persists, scintigraphy can be a more sensitive indicator of treatment response than clinical symptoms, chest radiographs, and pulmonary function tests [21]. Gallium-67 scintigraphy has also been proposed for the early detection of interstitial pneumonitis associated with certain therapies (bleomycin etc.). Diffuse pulmonary uptake in patients receiving immunosuppressant drugs is suggestive of Pneumocystis carinii infection. Pneumocystis carinii pneumonia is also the most common AIDS-related opportunistic infection. Gallium-67 is used as an index to stage interstitial lung disorders together with other activity markers in idiopathic pulmonary fibrosis,

extrinsic allergic alveolitis, pneumoconiosis, tuberculosis and other granulomatoses and collagen vascular diseases.

Whatever the clinical indication among those presented here, the pathological uptake of gallium-67 is clearly delineated from the vascular and normal tissue background as well as from bone marrow most of the time. Nevertheless, technical considerations are as important as carefully preparing the patient, especially in cases of diffuse nodular lesions poorly distinguished from neighboring structures.

DTPA scintigraphy

Several pathological factors can damage the membrane of the respiratory units and can lead to a disturbance of gas exchange. In order to prevent or reduce the degree of damage to this membrane the lesions should be recognized as early as possible for early initiation of adequate treatment.

Many methods have been proposed for the

assessment of the status of the pulmonary membranes (pulmonary radiography, thoracic scanning, spirography, diffusion testing, determination of the alveolo-arterial O_2 gradient) including the technetium-99m DTPA pulmonary clearance test.

Histological bases of DTPA clearance

The structure and function of the respiratory tract and alveolar-capillary region are described in detail in Chapter "Physiopathological bases", first two paragraphes. Nevertheless some specific points concerning DTPA clearance must be stressed.

The respiratory units (terminal bronchioli and alveoli) are involved in gas exchange.

The alveolar-capillary membrane is formed of two cell layers separated by an interstitial space.

The epithelial layer in the alveoli is formed principally of two types of cells (pneumocytes types I and II) lying on a basal membrane. These cells are interconnected by intercellular bridges composed of several layers of proteins.

The capillary endothelial layer contains endothelial cells lying also on a basal membrane.

The alveolar and capillary basal membranes are composed of bilaminar lipid structures containing proteins, glycoproteins and cholesterol.

Molecules with strong liposolubility pass across the membranes more readily than hydrophilic molecules. In addition, small hydrosoluble molecules pass across the capillary wall ten times as rapidly as across the alveolar wall. These molecules pass through the membranes mainly at the level of the intercellular pores. The diameter of these pores is 0.8 to 1 nm in the alveolar epithelium and 4 to 8 nm in the capillary endothelium. Additionally, the alveolar lumen is lined with the surfactant produced by type II pneumocytes. To some extent this liquid film impairs the passage of hydrosoluble molecules from the alveolar lumen to the vascular lumen.

The interstitial space is more or less developed in various parts of the lungs and it contains immuno-competent cells, supportive tissue and lymphatic vessels, the importance of which varies depending on the territory supplied by them.

The vector necessary for the study of the integrity of the alveolar-capillary membrane should be stable, chemically inert, electrically neutral, hydrophilic and passively diffusible. DTPA (diethylenetriamine pent-acetate) has the characteristics required for this exploration, its molecular weight being 492 daltons and its diameter 0.6 nm.

The diffusion of DTPA labeled with ^{99m}Tc across the membrane is proportional to the difference in the concentrations in the alveolar space and capillary space, and to the area of the membrane involved in the exchange. In clinical practice the constant of technetium-99m DTPA is measured from the monoexponential curve derived from the time/radioactivity curve based on dynamic recording.

Physiology of the pulmonary clearance of technetium-99m DTPA

The kinetics of aerosols are detailed in Chapter "Physiopathological bases". As the aim is to study the alveolar-capillary clearance of DTPA, a homogeneous peripheral deposition has to be achieved. Therefore, DTPA aerosol has to be administered with a nebulizer giving a MMAD below 2 μm. This is usually achieved by using jet nebulizers at a high flow rate (6 to 9 l/mn). Nevertheless, in certain pathological conditions the central accumulation of the radioactivity may be greater due to impairment of peripheral penetration. In extreme situations, poorly or non-ventilated regions may have insufficient penetration of the radioaerosol be able to study the pulmonary clearance of technetium-99m DTPA.

The bronchial clearance of the radioaerosol takes several hours and is due mainly to the mucociliary mechanism. The pulmonary clearance of DTPA takes place mainly through the bloodstream (clearance is reduced to half its value after obstruction of the pulmonary artery, and elimination of the particles is through the bronchial vessels). Clearance through the lymphatic vessels plays a negligible role (2-3%).

The passage of technetium-99m DTPA molecules from the aerated lumen of the alveoli to the vascular lumen occurs mainly through the intercellular pores of the alveolar epithelium. Many factors can affect the rate of transmembrane passage. The body position of the patient during the test and respiratory rhythm can modify the pulmonary clearance in various areas. In the sitting position the clearance is faster in the apical areas than at the base of the lungs. This pattern is reversed in the supine position. Deep inspiration increases the rate of pulmonary clearance of DTPA, while polypnea with reduced tidal volume or increased inspiratory flow exerts an opposite effect. Increased liquid volume of the surfactant also reduces the pulmonary clearance of DTPA (in view of this, clearance tests should not be performed shortly after bronchiolo-alveolar lavage).

Methods for study of the pulmonary clearance of technetium-99m DTPA

Various methods have been described in the literature, but here we discuss only the method which is most often used and which allows the integration of various parameters which potentially influence the results of the study.

Initially a static image recorded on the posterior face of the thorax (background activity) is obtained 30-60 seconds before the beginning of radioaerosol inhalation. Then nebulization of ^{99m}Tc-DTPA is begun to obtain particles of one micron size (20-30 mCi in a nebulizer) for 2-3 minutes with the patient's back to the gamma camera, preferably in the supine position. The respiratory rate (12-18 per minute) and the tidal volume should be normal. The inhalation of the aerosol is terminated after recording 1500-2000 cps over the lungs.

From the beginning of radioaerosol inhalation, recording is carried out at intervals of 30 or 60 seconds over 20 minutes. At the end of this recording perfusion scintigraphy on the posterior face of the thorax is carried out, injecting 2-3 mCi of technetium-99m MAA. In order to obtain activity/time curves, regions of interest are chosen in the upper and lower halves of each lung. The background activity image obtained initially is subtracted from each image recorded. The half-life or the percentage of the diminution per minute is calculated in the first 7 or 10 minutes after the peak of the monoexponential curve. The half-life is reduced and the percentage decrease of the radioactivity per minute is increased when the pulmonary clearance of DTPA is accelerated.

Qualitative analysis of the ventilation (distribution and penetration of the radioaerosol) and perfusion (perfusion defects) are useful for the interpretation of the obtained values. The choice of the regions of interest should take into account these images. In particular, the excessive accumulation of radioactivity in the bronchi should not be included in the regions of interest chosen for the calculations, since this can give false results. However, for reliable results the nebulizer should deliver the technetium-99m DTPA aerosol with a labeling purity exceeding 95%. In fact, TcO_4^- passes 4-5 times more rapidly across the pulmonary barrier than technetium-99m DTPA. The dissociation of ^{99m}Tc from DTPA can be demonstrated objectively by visualization of the thyroid on the images of ventilation function. Chromatographic analysis of the parent solution (placed in the nebulizer) and of the aerosol (obtained at the outlet of the nebulizer) makes possible more precise quantitative determination of the radiochemical purity of the radiotracer, especially with a more accurate determination of the content of TcO_4^- (which has a high diffusion capacity) and TcO_2, which is colloidal and cannot pass across the alveolocapillary membrane. The choice of the generator, the concentration of stannous chloride and the nebulizer can influence these different parameters.

In non-smoker control subjects, the half-life is 60 ± 15 minutes and the percentage decrease per minute is $1.21 \pm 0.5\%$. In smokers the pulmonary clearance of DTPA is accelerated by a factor of 2-3 times and is normalized about one month after discontinuation of smoking.

Scintigraphy for the evaluation of mucociliary clearance

Introduction

Measurement of mucociliary clearance requires following a radiolabeled tracer that is deposited by aerosol. The tracer should be deposited on the bronchi from the second to fifth generation. For the further generations, other mechanisms are involved in lung clearance. The size of the radiolabeled particles should be between 4 and 8 μm, to allow deposition in the main bronchi.

Several nebulizers can be used to generate radiolabeled aerosol, according to nebulization parameters, particle size and the isotope.

Ultrasonic nebulizers or jet nebulizers produce an aerosol which can be inhaled during a single forced breath or controlled breathing.

There are several suitable particles available: lucite, manganese dioxide, serum albumin, resin or polystyrene; another way is to use the patient's red blood cells [26, 27].

Numerous isotopes have been proposed: 38 F, 51 Cr, 54 Mn, 59 Fe, 131 I, 198 Au. The choice of the isotope depends on labeling problems and the duration of the examination. Because of availability, cost and characteristics of the isotope, [99m]Tc(T = 6 h) is the most often used for short study and [131]I (T = 8 d) for longer ones.

Our technique can be used in any Deparment of Nuclear Medicine; it allows analysis of overall mucociliary clearance. It can be modified in accordance with the availability of the equipment and the aim of the study. [99m]Tc radiolabeled red blood cells

Fig. 7. Image processing of left lung recorded on posterior face. *Lb* left bronchi; *Ll* left lung

Fig. 8. Initial deposition is defined as follows:

$$= \frac{3+4+5}{1+2+3+4+5}$$

It reflects the control over peripheral deposition. The examination can be analyzed if the index is above 70%; if it is below, the examination must be excluded [3]

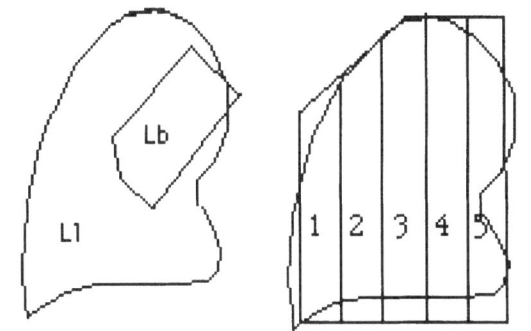

are inhaled during 10 min controlled breathing; they are deposited on the main bronchi, and followed for 90 min.

The aerosol

Five milliliters of blood are drawn on anticoagulant; red blood cells are washed to avoid adhesion, sensitized with stannous pyrophosphate and labeled with ^{99m}Tc.

Production of the aerosol

Specific activity of red cells is 185 MBq/ml (5 mCi/ ml); they are nebulized by a Venturi generator and breathing is controlled through a mouthpiece for about 10 mn.

Image acquisition

Images are obtained from a posterior view of the seated patient. Two hundred ten pictures, 30 sec long, are recorded over 90 mn after completing the aerosol.

Image analysis

Four regions of interest are defined (fig. 7) corresponding to the main bronchi and the lung.
    Analysis of curves:
    – from the initial curves:
        • background subtraction,
        • correction of physical decay,
        • subtraction of bronchial activity,
    – from pulmonary activity: normalization according to bronchial areas (constant), and pulmonary areas (variable, drawn on the screen).

Normal semiology

Deposition index

Whatever the technique used to produce the aerosol, the tracer must be deposited on the main bronchi. This is essential for the interpretation of the examination. Analysis of the examination begins with a check on the

penetration of the aerosol and the computation of a deposition index.
    Numerous indices have been suggested; we use one that corresponds to anatomic criteria described in figure 8. The lung is divided into five areas of equal width.
    Initial deposition is defined as follows:

$$= \frac{3+4+5}{1+2+3+4+5}$$

It reflects the control over peripheral deposition. The examination can be analyzed if the index is above 70%; if it is below, the examination must be excluded [3].
    The sedimentation of red blood cells is mainly on main bronchi, but also in the lung:
    The solution of this two compartmental model (fig. 9), produces the following equations:

During deposition of aerosol:

$$a_1(t) = A_1 \left(1 - e^{-k_1 t}\right)$$
$$a_2(t) = A_2 + B_2 e^{-k_1 t} + C_2 e^{-k_2 t}$$

constants are expressed as below:

$$A_1 = \frac{\alpha}{k_1}$$

$$A_2 = \frac{\alpha + \beta}{k_2}, \quad B_2 = -\frac{\alpha}{k_1 + k_2}, \quad C_2 = \frac{k_1(\alpha + \beta) - k_2 \beta}{(k_2 - k_1) k_2}$$

α and β are the curves of the tangents from the pulmonary and bronchial curves presented on figure 4.

*After deposition of the aerosol
(time of the examination)*

$$a_1(t) = A_1 e^{-k_1 t}$$
$$a_2(t) = A_2 e^{-k_1 t} + B_2 e^{-k_2 t}$$

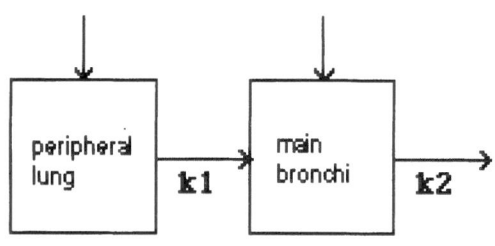

9

Fig. 9. Modelization. a1 (t) bronchial activity; a2 (t) pulmonary activity. *k1*, *k 2* constant of transfer

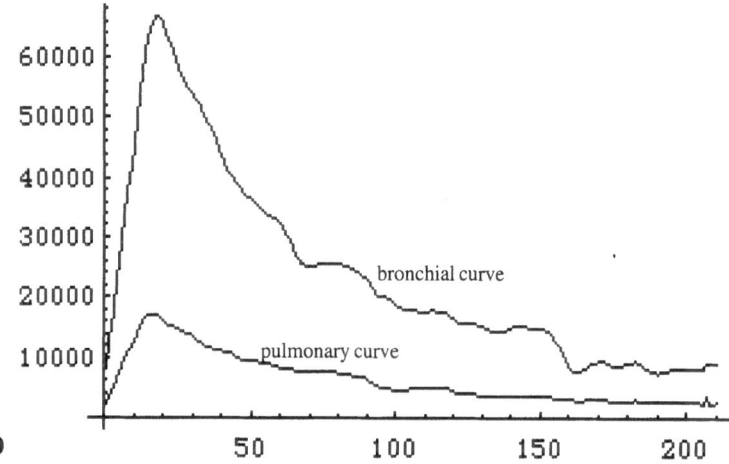

10

Fig. 10. Variation of radioactivity over 90 mn

Table 2. Normal muco ciliary clearance in 10 healthy non smoker subjects

		60 mn	90 mn
Main bronchi	Right	m = 57.6%	m = 63.4%
		σ = 7.5%	σ = 7.3%
	Left	m = 55.8%	m = 61.0%
		σ = 6.7%	σ = 6.8%
Peripheral lung	Right	m = 49.9%	m = 53.4%
		σ = 6.4%	σ = 7.6%
	Left	m = 46.0%	m = 56.4%
		σ = 5.6%	σ = 9.0%

$$A_1 = A_1(\max)$$

$$A_2 = \frac{k_1 A_1(\max)}{k_2 - k_1}, \quad B_2 = \frac{k_2(k_2 - k_1)A_1(\max)A_2(\max)}{k_2 - k_1}$$

Presentation of results (fig. 10)

The picture at the end of the aerosol allows the evaluation of the amount of the deposit and its homogeneity.

Following the pictures at 0, 30, 60, 90 mn shows good elimination of the radioactivity (fig. 11).

Data processing

Clearance is defined as the percentage of the activity at 1 hour and 11/2 hours, from the maximum of the deposit at the end of the aerosol; clearances are defined for the main bronchi and the lung (table 2).

For control subjects, normal values are:
– left deposit indicator: m = 82.5%, s = 4.5%
– right deposit indicator: m = 81.2%, s = 4.7%

Of course it is possible to use more elaborate mathematical methods to identify the curves as a function of the exponential model proposed.

Pathologic semiology

During nebulization, aerosol deposition may be heterogeneous, especially in asthma or bronchiectasis. When mucociliary clearance is impaired, activity curves lose their biexponential character and become a

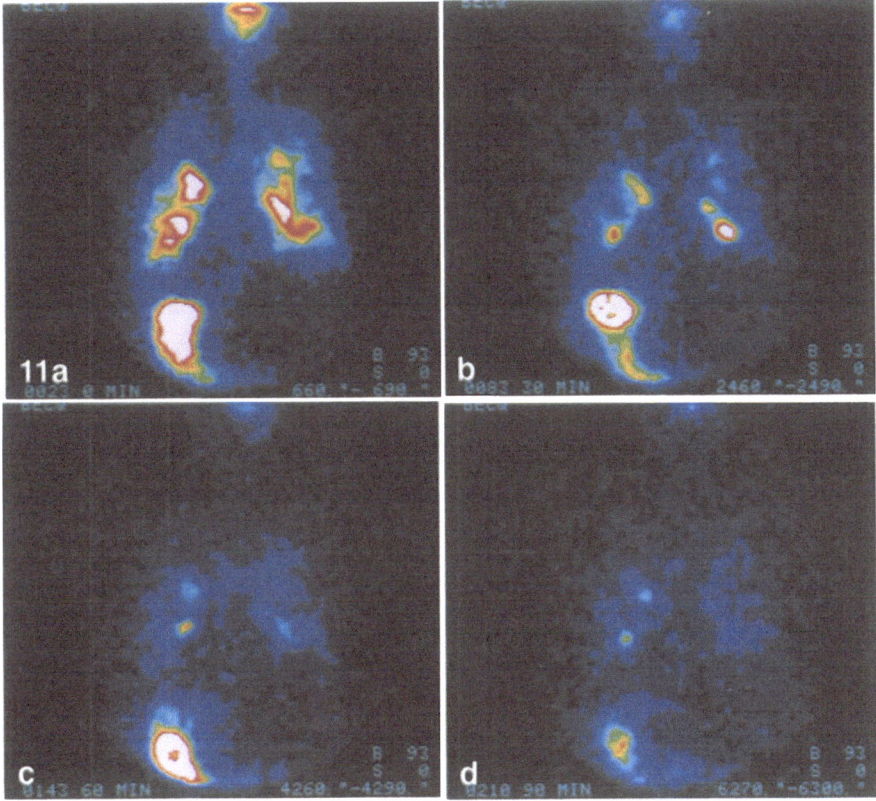

Fig. 11. Normal mucociliary clearance recorded on posterior face 0, 30, 60 and minutes after the end of inhalation

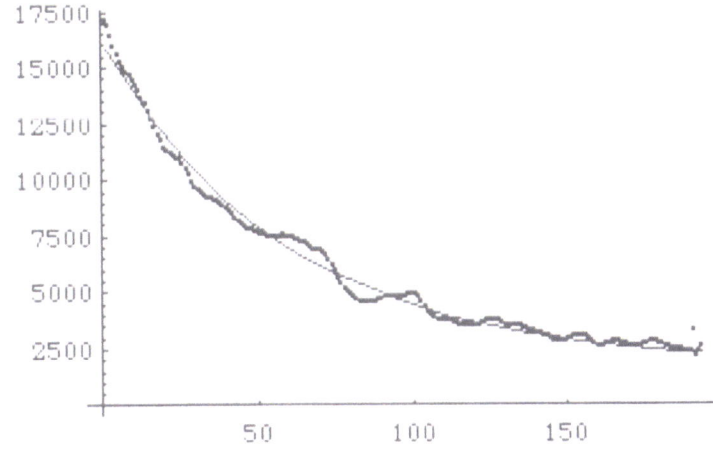

Fig. 12. Identification of the clearance phase of the previous pulmonary curve. Maximal activity 17,201 beats.

$$a_1(t) = 1757 + 14352 \; \exp\left(-t\big/60\right)$$

Clearance at 1 hour -78%

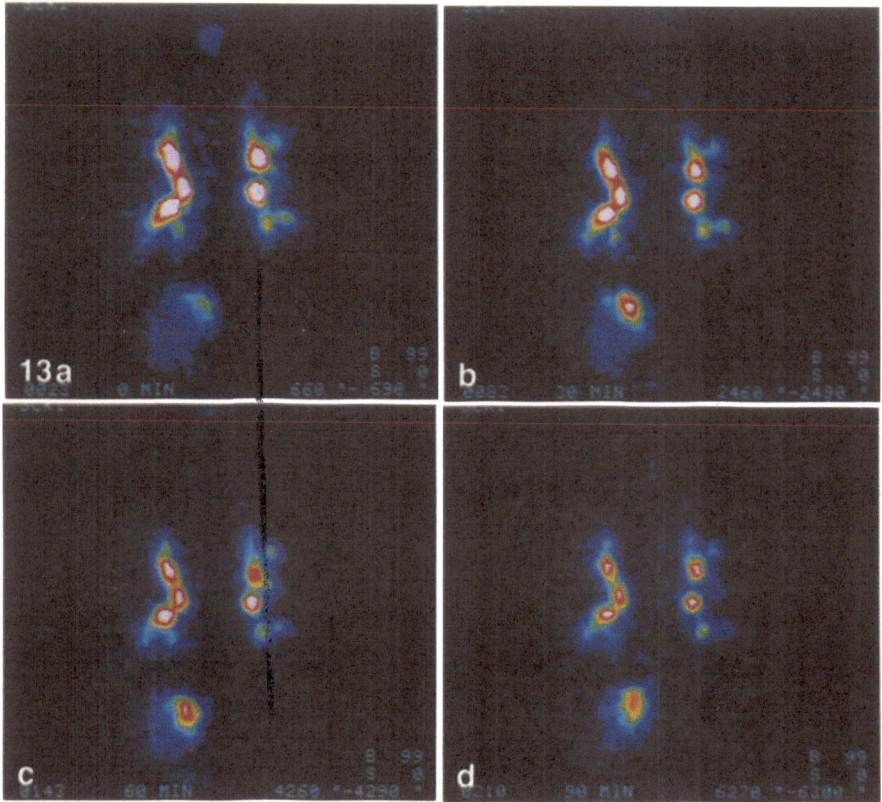

Fig.13. Impaired mucociliary clearance recorded on posterior face 0, 30, 60 and 90 minutes after the end of inhalation in a patient suffering from cystic fibrosis

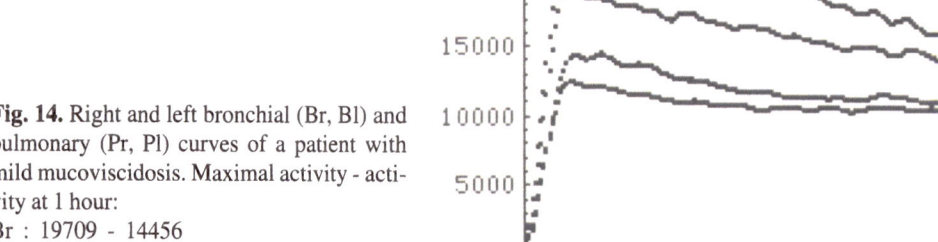

Fig. 14. Right and left bronchial (Br, Bl) and pulmonary (Pr, Pl) curves of a patient with mild mucoviscidosis. Maximal activity - activity at 1 hour:
Br : 19709 - 14456
Bl : 25790 - 15975
Pr : 12366 - 10375

straight line, showing a reduction in clearance of the main bronchi.

Clearance is decreased and values may drop to about 20% at 1 hour (fig. 13).

References

1. Wellman HN (1986) Pulmonary Thromboembolism : Current status. Report on the Role of Nuclear Medicine. Sem Nucl Med 16 : 236-274

2. Taplin GV, Johnson DE, Dore EK et al (1964) Suspensions of radioalbumin aggregates for photoscanning the liver, spleen, lung and other organs. J Nucl Med 5 : 259-275

3. Taplin GV (1979) The History of Lung Imaging with Radionuclides. Sem Nucl Med 9 : 178-185

4. Nielson PE, Kirchner PT, Gerber FH (1977) Oblique views in lung perfusion scanning : clinical utility and limitations. J Nucl Med 18 : 967-972

5. De Nardo GL, Goodwin DA, Ravasini R et al (1970) The ventilatory lung scan in the diagnosis of pulmonary embolism. N Engl J Med 282 : 1334-1336

6. Alderson PO, Lee H, Summer WR et al (1979) Comparison of xenon-133 washout and singlebreath imaging for the detection of ventilation abnormalities. J Nucl Med 20 : 917-922

7. Alpert NM, Mckusick KA, Correia JA et al (1976) Initial assessment of a simple functional image of ventilation. J Nucl Med 17 : 88-92

8. Rawbone RG (1976) Evaluation of and integrated ^{133}Xe regional pulmonary-function analyzer. J Nucl Med 17 : 337-344

9. Fazio F, Jones T (1975) Assessment of regional ventilation by continuous inhalation of radioactive krypton-81m. Br Med J 3 : 673-676

10. Schor RA, Shames DM, Weber PM et al (1978) Regional ventilation studies with [81m]Kr and [133]Xe : a comparative analysis. J Nucl Med 19 : 348-353

11. Royston D, Minty BD (1984) A single separator to generate half micron aqueous particles for lung imaging. Br J Radiol 57 : 223-228

12. Burch WM, Sullivan PJ, McLaren CJ (1986) Technegas — a new ventilation agent for lung scanning. Nuclear Medicine Communications 7 : 865-871

13. Hoffer P (1980) Gallium : Mechanisms. J Nucl Med 21 : 282-285

14. Edwards CL, Hayes RL (1969) Tumor scanning with gallium-67 citrate. J Nucl Med 10 : 103-105

15. Bekerman C, Hoffer PB, Bitran JD, Gupta RG (1980) Gallium-67 citrate imaging studies of the lung. Sem Nucl Med 10 : 286-301

16. Klech H, Köhn H, Huppmann M, Pohl W (1987) Thoracic maging with gallium-67. Eur J Nucl Med 13 : S24-S36

17. Vallabhajosula S, Goldsmith SJ, Lipszyc H, Chahinian AP, Ohnuma T (1983) Gallium-transferrin and gallium-lactoferrin binding to tumor cells. Specific versus nonspecific glycoprotein-cell interaction. Eur J Nucl Med 8 : 354-357

18. Chen DCP, Hung GL, Levine A, Siegel ME (1986) Correlation of gallium uptake and degre of malignancy in non-Hodgkin's lymphoma (abstr). J Nucl Med 27 : 1031

19. Meideros LJ, Picker LJ, Horning SJ, Warnke RA (1988) Transferrin receptor expression by non-Hodgkin's lymphomas. Correlation with morphologic grade and survival. Cancer 61 : 1844-1851

20. Kaplan WD (1990) Editorial : residual mass and negative gallium scintigraphy in treated lymphoma : when is the gallium scan really negative ? J Nucl Med 31 : 369-371

21. Baughman RP, Fernandez M, Bosken CH, Mantil J, Hurtubise P (1984) Am Rev Respir Dis 129 : 676-681

22. Coates G and O'Brodovich H (1986) Measurement of pulmonary epithelial permeability with ^{99m}Tc-DTPA aerosol. Sem Nucl Med : 275-284

23. Dusser D, Minty B, Collignon MA, Hinge D, Barritault L, Huchon G (1986) Regional respiratory clearance of aerosolized ^{99m}Tc-DTPA : Posture and smoking effects. J Appl Physiol 60 : 2000-2006

24. Evander E, Wollmer P, Jonson B, Lachmann B (1987) Pulmonary clearance of inhaled ^{99m}Tc-DTPA : effects of surfactant depletion by lung lavage. J Appl Physiol 1611-1614

25. Jones JG, Royston D and Minty BD (1983) Changes in alveolar-capillary barrier function in animals and humans. Am Rev Respir Dis 127 : S51-S59

26. Rühle KH, Köhler D, Fischer J, Matthhys H (1979) Measurement of Mucociliairy Clearance with ^{99m}Tc-Tagget Erythrocytes. Prog Resp Res 11, 117-126

27. LaffiteJJ, Coequyt S, Duhamel A, Lemaire P, Mazzuca M (1984) Mise au point de techniques simples d'exploration de l'épuration mucociliaire. Rev Mal Resp 1 : 394

28. Agnew JE, Pavia D, Clarke SW (1968) Mucus Claerance from peripheral and central airways of asympomatic smokers. Bull Eur Physiopath Resp 22 : 263-267

29. Mezey RJ, Cohn MA, Fernandez RJ (1978) Mucociliary transport in allergic patients with antigen-induced bronchospasm. Am Rev Respir Dis 118 : 677-684

Practical notions for carrying out nuclear medicine examination

JL Baulieu

This chapter examines the practical process of an examination using nuclear medicine, i.e. patient referral, appointment for nuclear imaging, preparation of radio isotope, radio pharmaceutical administration, imaging, interpretation, medical report and cost evaluation of manipulation.

The main objectives are to explain how a nuclear medicine department works and what happens to the patient: timing, risk, discomfort, information, co-operation (fig. 1).

A short paragraph will be devoted to dosimetry and radioprotection.

Referral and appointment

A general rule is that every nuclear medicine examination is performed on the basis of a written referral. This is essential for an appropriate protocol schedule and a relevant report. It is also indispensable that the patient brings a recent chest X-ray.

The appointment is made by telephone with the patient or the referring physician. The diagnosis of pulmonary embolism is an emergency and the scintigraphy is performed without delay. When possible a permanent service is organized to come to the emergency department at any time.

The examination of in-patients is performed during hospitalization according to tracer availability.

The follow-up examinations can be scheduled over a longer period of time and usually performed as an out-patient or during day-hospitalisation.

Radioisotope availability and radiopharmaceutical preparation

The ^{99m}Tc radiolabeled tracers are easily available.

They are delivered in a kit containing the molecule and a reduction agent, most often tin chloride (Sn Cl$_2$), in a lyophilized form. The labeling is simply achieved by adding a freshly eluted technetium solution and shaking for 3 to 5 min. The radiopharmaceutical solution is drawn up into a syringe and the activity is checked in a well counting detector.

^{133}Xe, ^{67}Ga and ^{131}I can be obtained to order.

The delivery is usually 1 to 3 days. The tracer is the element form and the radiotracer is delivered ready for use. However the activity must always be checked before patient administration.

^{81m}Kr is eluted from a ^{81}Rb generator (see Chapter "Physical and technical bases"). As ^{81}Rb half-life is only 4.7 hr, the generator has to be delivered on the day of examination. Moreover ^{81m}Kr itself has a 13 sec. half-life. Elution yield must be high, about 2 l.mn^{-1}, in order to replace the gas lost by physical decay and expiration.

^{123}I has also to be delivered on the day of the examination

Only the meta iodo benzyl guanidine I-123 (^{123}I

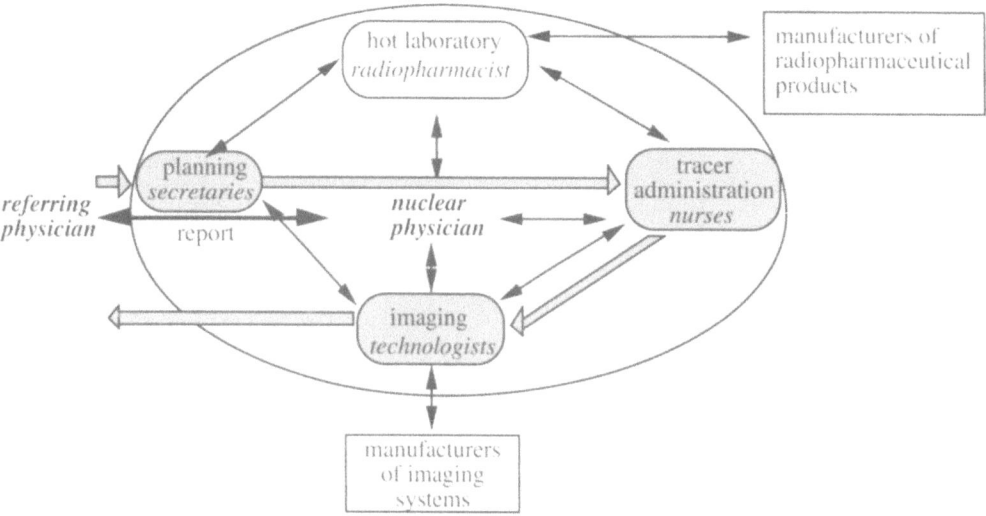

Fig. 1. Nuclear medicine department. Structure and organisation. ⟷ informations exchange ⇨ patient experience

MIBG) and the iodo amphetamine I-123 (^{123}I AMP) are commercially available in a kit form. However the labeling is noticeably more complicated than Tc labeling and the cost of ^{123}I is higher.

^{111}In is used for molecular and cellular labeling

It has to be ordered for each application. The delivery is about 1 to 3 days. The ^{111}In radiolabeled antibodies are ready for injection on delivery or prepared on site according a simple procedure of ^{111}In and antibody solution mixing. The ^{111}In radiolabeled somatostatin analogs (^{111}In SMS) are only available in a limited number of European countries. For cell labeling, ^{111}In is delivered as ^{111}In oxinate. Autologous cell labeling requires patient blood sampling, cell separation, labeling and purification.

These operations are carried out under sterile conditions and with gentle handling in order to preserve cell viability. The labeled cells are resuspended in the patient's own plasma before reinjection.

It is desirable that these tasks, i.e. ordering and management of radioelements, radiopharmaceutical labeling, purification and control, are performed under the responsibility and control of a qualified radiopharmacist.

Tracer administration

The patient receives the tracer in a special injection or inhalation room. Sometimes, when the input or early distribution has to be recorded, the tracer is administered to the patient already positioned in the detection field of the camera. The operator may be a nuclear physician, a nurse or a technologist. Tracer injection is performed using a lead shielded syringe to minimize operator hand irradiation. The tracer is directly injected into an antebrachial vein or through a small previously inserted catheter equipped with a 3-way tap.

Inhalation requires a closed circuit inhalation device fitted with a filter in order to avoid room contamination. The patient inhales the radio-pharmaceutical through a mouth adaptor or a mask. In the latter case the patient's head is placed in an aspirating hood communicating with the outside through a filter. Inhalation requires the patient's cooperation which is not necessary for injection.

Tracer administration is well tolerated and does not entail any risk. Allergic manifestations are very rare but theoretically possible, namely after glycopeptide, peptide analogs (SMS) and antibody administration. In any case, it must be considered a rule to minimize the administered tracer radioactivity, in order to reduce patient and staff irradiation (see paragraph "Irradiation - Radioprotection").

Imaging time

The imaging time depends on the radiotracer metabolism and the radioisotope period. In some cases, the transit kinetics are informative, i.e. input, equilibrium and clearance. Ventilation and esophageal

Table 1. Imaging time

Examination	Radiopharmaceutical	Imaging time
1. Early imaging		
Perfusion	^{99m}Tc macroaggregates or microspheres	5mn
Ventilation	^{99m}Tc DTPA, ^{133}Xe, ^{81m}Kr	during and 20 mn after tracer inhalation
2. Imaging within hours		
Bone scan	^{99m}Tc MDP	3 hr
3. Imaging within days		
Inflammation	^{67}Ga	2 d
Thyroid metastases	^{131}I	2-3 d
Infection	^{111}In polynuclears	1 d
Immunoscintigraphy	^{111}In antibodies	3 d

transit are examples. In these cases, the activity is recorded by dynamic imaging, during and after tracer administration (see paragraph "Tracer administration"). In other cases, organ or lesion uptake is informative: the optimal imaging time is reached when the uptake background ratio is maximal. The increase in uptake background ratio is due to progressive local tracer accumulation combined with circulating tracer elimination by renal or hepatic clearance. Another factor affecting the optimal imaging time is the absolute activity count decrease, the rate of which depends on the radio-element half-life.

Schematically, three types of timing can be considered:

– early post-injection imaging: macroaggregate or microsphere perfusion scintigraphy, the tracer is trapped in the lung at the first pass through the lungs and the extrapulmonary background is practically negligible;

– imaging in the hours following injection: imaging with phosphonate-^{99m}Tc (^{99m}Tc MDP), ^{123}I MIBG, ^{123}I AMP is performed early (3 or 6 hours) after injection and late (24 hours) after injection. The absolute activity subsequently becomes too low due to the physical decay;

– imaging in the days following injection: the relatively long half-lives of ^{67}Ga, ^{111}In, ^{131}I allow imaging time up to 3 - 5 days.

The usual imaging times for some routine scintigraphic studies are summarized in table 1.

Imaging support

Imaging support has two functions - image storage and image transmission. They are different according to whether the image is analogical or digital.

Analogical images require photography of the oscilloscope screen on film or paper (see Chapter "Physical and technical bases"). The film is a high quality, lasting image support. However it requires manual developing and is relatively expensive. Polaroid® films offer the convenience of instant developing. However they do not have the sensitivity of the classic emulsion films and image quality rapidly fades with time.

Digital images are stored on a magnetic tape, a numeric magnetic hard or floppy disk, or an optical disk. The advantage of the optical disk is the high storage capacity and the short access time. A 128 x 128 pixel with 16 bits per pixel to code matrix takes up 262144 bits or 32768 octets (1 octets = 8 bits). A 80 megaoctect (1 megaoctet = 1 Mo = 10^6 octets) capacity disk has a storage capacity of 2,424 [128 x 128] matrices or 150 [64 x (64 x 64)] tomographic acquisitions.

The image, sequence of images or tomographic image reconstructions are displayed on a TV monitor. It is reproduced on a color or black and white videoprinter, or directly transferred from the computer onto a digital printer. The printer is capable of printing on paper (ink impression or heat sensitive paper) and

Table 2. Cost evaluation of manipulation and costs of radio-pharmaceutical products. Z value is 8.1 FF (February 1993)

	Cost evaluation of manipulation	Radiopharmaceutical cost (FF)
Perfusion		
^{99m}Tc macroaggregates	100 Z	1420
^{133}Xe solution	150 Z	800
Ventilation		
^{99m}Tc DTPA	150 Z	780
^{133}Xe gas	150 Z	800
Bone scan (^{99m}TcMDP)	150 Z	1030
^{123}I MIBG	150 Z	1370
^{131}I diagnosis	260 Z	420
^{131}I therapy	100 Z	
^{67}Ga	150 Z	1580
^{111}In antibody immunoscintigraphy	150 Z	950

on photopolaroid, black and white film or colour slides.

Interpretation – Report

A report of the examination must be written by the nuclear physician on the day of examination, and sent with the most significant imaging document to the referring physician.

Reading and interpretation are performed on good quality original documents or directly from the data processing system display.

The report should include the identities of the patient and referring physician, date and file reference number. The protocol should be summarized with tracer, radioactivity administered, patient preparation, imaging time (see above), imaging duration and modalities (see Chapter "Physical and technical bases", paragraph " Isotopes and radio-activity"), and data processing (see Chapter "Physical and technical bases", paragraph " Isotopes and radio-activity"). A description of the visual examination and index or parameter data should be given. A conclusion should summarize the scintigraphic observations, possibly compared with previous examinations, and suggest the diagnostic interpretation.

Report editing is made easy and fast with the help of word or data processing, including a framework and current items.

Act costing

The costing is an evaluation of the cost of carrying out an examination. It takes into account the duration of the examination, the type of detector required, and data processing. It does not included the cost of the radiotracer. Table 2 gives examples of costing scale applied in a French Nuclear Medicine department. It has to be noted that the global cost is subject to variation according to the protocol of the examination, the number of examinations performed with a radiopharmaceutical kit and the ^{99m}Tc generator cost price.

Irradiation – radioprotection

Dosimetry – units

During passage through matter radiation deposits energy by direct or indirect ionization (see Chapter "Physical and technical bases", § " Isotopes and radio-activity"). The ionization of atoms and molecules produces structural modifications of biological material which may be responsible for cell death, cancerisation and metabolic or genetic changes.

The deposited energy is measured by the absorbed dose in rad or gray (Gy): 1 rad = 100 ergs/gramme = 10^{-2} joules/kg. 1 Gy = 100 rads = 1 joule/kg.

The biological effects depend on the absorbed dose

Table 3. Equivalent irradiation dose for routine scintigraphic examinations

Examination	Radiotracer	Equivalent dose(mSv)	
		Lung	Whole body
Perfusion	[99m]Tc macroaggregates (110 MBq)	4.5	< 0.03
Ventilation	[99m]Tc DTPA aerosol (110 MBq)	1.5	0.5
	[133]Xe gas (110MBq)	1.5	< 0.03
	[81m]Kr gas (185MBq)	0.2	< 0.03
Metabolism	[123]I MIBG (130 MBq)	0.2	0.3
Inflammation	[67]Ga (110 MBq)	–	
	[99m]Tc J01A (110 MBq)	0.75	
Immunoscintigraphy	[111]In Ab (185 MBq)	–	27
Bone scan	[99m]Tc MDP (740 MBq)	–	1.5

and on the radiation type. The equivalent dose is obtained by multiplying the absorbed dose by the radiation quality factor.

The quality factor is 1 for X, γ, and ß ray, and 20 for particles and neutrons. This means that for a given absorbed dose, the biological effects are 20 times greater with particles or neutrons than with X, γ, or ß radiations. The unit of dose equivalent is the rem corresponding to the rad and the sievert (Sv) corresponding to the Gy (1Gy = 100 rad, 1Sv = 100 rem). The dose equivalent is usually expressed in mSv (1mSv = 10^{-3} Sv).

Patient irradiation

Table 3 lists the equivalent irradiation doses for some current scintigraphic examinations. It shows two types of examination, the first type with lung uptake or transit giving no or low extrapulmonary irradiation, i.e. ventilation and perfusion examination; and the second with whole body metabolism which is responsible for a higher whole body irradiation dose i.e. gallium scan, immunoscintigraphy and bone scan. The equivalent dose values are to be compared with the annual natural irradiation dose, and with the irradiation dose delivered by one chest X-ray radiography, which are about 1 mSv. Broadly speaking, the irradiation dose due to scintigraphic examination is between the natural and radiological irradiation dose. It has to be noted that, unlike radiological examinations, patient irradiation does not depend on the number or duration of images.

Radioprotection

The aim of radioprotection is to keep public, workers', and patients' irradiation to the lowest level. Irradiation is due to external exposure and to possible internal contamination by ingestion or inhalation of radioactive substances.

The means of radioprotection are:
– dose limitation,
– controled zone,
– working rules.

The external exposure dose limit is set at up to 5 mSv per year for the public, and to 50 mSv per year for persons professionally exposed to radiation. The rate of irradiation must be less than 0.025 mSv/hr. The personal external radiation dose is checked by individual X- and γ-ray sensitive films. Film exposure is measured each month.

The internal contamination dose depends on the radioelement. For example, it is 2 MBq for [131]I. Internal contamination is detected and measured by urine radiotoxicology examination.

The controled zone is the area where unsealed radioactive sources are handled. The zone perimeter is marked by the controled zone sign (fig. 2). Access to the controled zone is limited to authorized persons. A bylaw must be posted and known by everybody who works in the controled zone.

The working rules are essential to minimize the irradiation dose, i.e. fast handling, use of shields, distance from sources. The radioactive sources must never be pipeted by mouth. The work rooms must be

Fig. 2. Controled zone sign

aired at a rate of 5 room volumes per hour. This is specially important when performing studies with radiolabeled gas and aerosol. Such rule observation results in safe working conditions. However it is essential to keep in mind that radiation hazards have no lower threshold. Radiation exposure must be justified in any given case by patient benefit. Protection has to be more and more optimized and the activity of the radiotracer must be limited to the lowest level.

Pulmonary embolism

F Baulieu and P Diot

The incidence of pulmonary embolism in the United States is estimated at 650,000 cases each year. About one third of these patients die [1]. On post mortem rates, diagnosis of pulmonary embolism is estimated between 10 and 20%. Prognosis depends upon the degree of pulmonary artery obstruction, appropriateness of treatment, long term chronic heart failure and risk of recurrence.

The sensitivity of clinical signs is less than 80%. Specificity is probably still lower, although it has not been precisely determined. Sensitivity is 80% for chest X-ray and 85% for hypoxemia. Nevertheless both of these criteria have low specificity. Electrocardiography reveals characteristic abnormalities in only 25% of patients [2].

Taking into account these parameters, it is obviously necessary to determine a strategy for accurate diagnosis of pulmonary embolism according to local facilities.

Place of isotopic techniques among diagnostic criteria

Although they are not not specific, first line investigations including clinical examination, chest X-ray, electrocardiography and blood gas analysis must be performed before any other investigations [3].

In cases where acute major pulmonary embolism is suspected on clinical signs such as syncope or acute right heart failure or in cases where anticoagulant therapy cannot be applied, angiography must be performed. Ventilation-perfusion scans would delay diagnosis [3].

In other cases perfusion scans or ventilation-perfusion scans can be included in the diagnostic strategies.

To be accurate a scan has to be performed within 48 hours of the acute phase. Moreover, it is considered that diagnosis of pulmonary embolism must be established or rejected within 24 hours after onset of symptoms. This is why it is important to consider the place and choice of nuclear medicine tests which depend upon local facilities.

Perfusion scans are the basis of isotopic investigations. They should be associated with ventilation scans in patients with a history of previous cardio-pulmonary disease. In view of difficulties of interpretation, some authors consider that scans are not indicated in such patients and they recommend angiograms. Nevertheless it has been demonstrated that the diagnostic value of ventilation-perfusion scans is not reduced by pre-existing cardiac or pulmonary disease [4, 5].

Ventilation-perfusion scans are also difficult to interpret in patients with history of previous pulmonary embolism who have not undergone a control scan. In such patients, images of hypo-perfusion have a predictive value only if located in new territories. This emphasizes the necessity of a control perfusion scan 1 to 2 months after the acute phase in patients with proven pulmonary embolism, even in patients who have not initially undergone a perfusion scan (figs. 1, 2) [6].

In pregnant women ventilation-perfusion scan can be performed without dosimetric risk for the fetus. If angiography subsequently appears to be necessary, it should be limited to 2 views. There are to date no

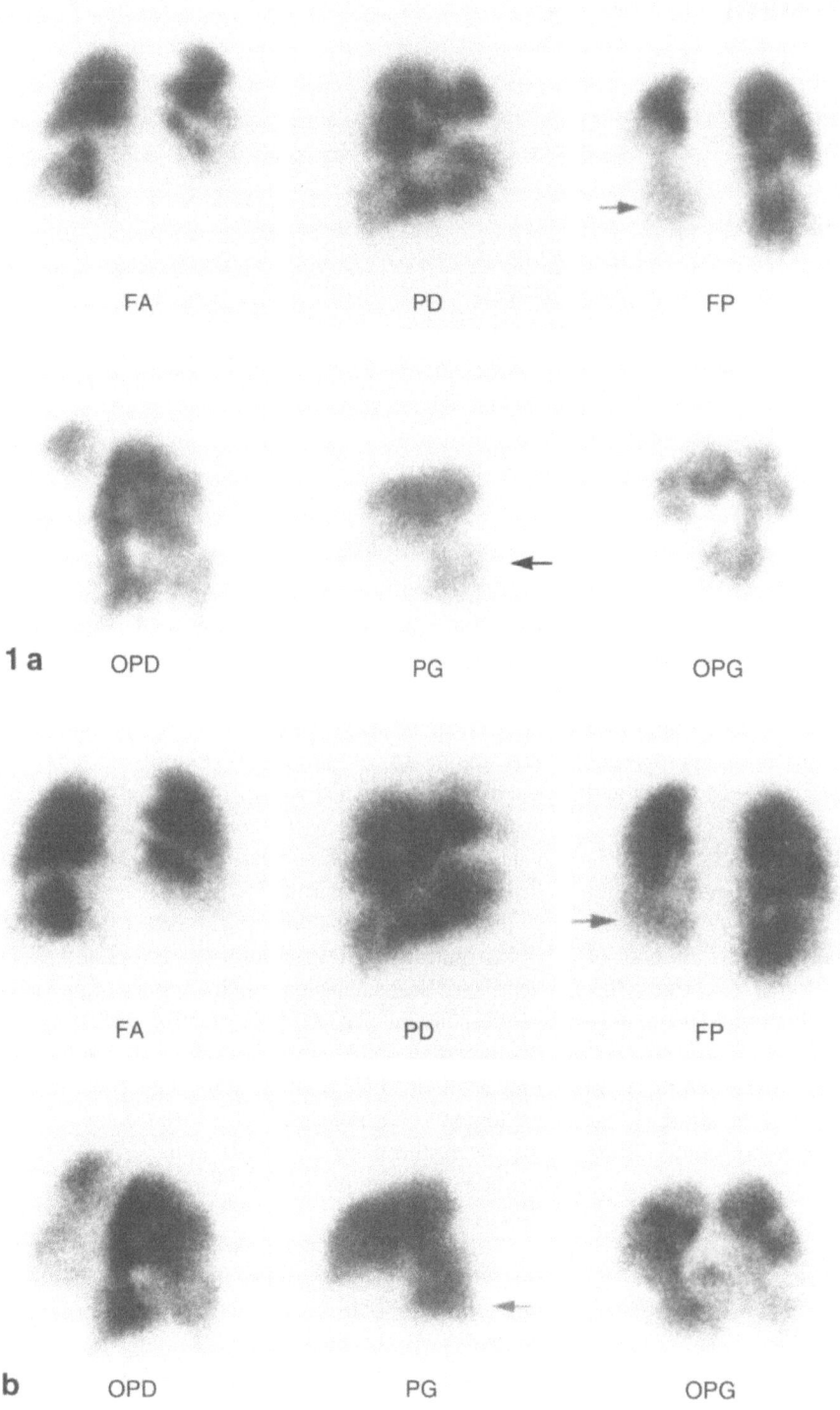

Fig. 1 a, b. Pulmonary embolism. **a** Initial perfusion scan shows extensive defects in both lungs. The defects predominate in the left lower lobe (→); **b** follow-up scan obtained 12 days later shows a substantial resolution of the defect in the left lower lobe (→)

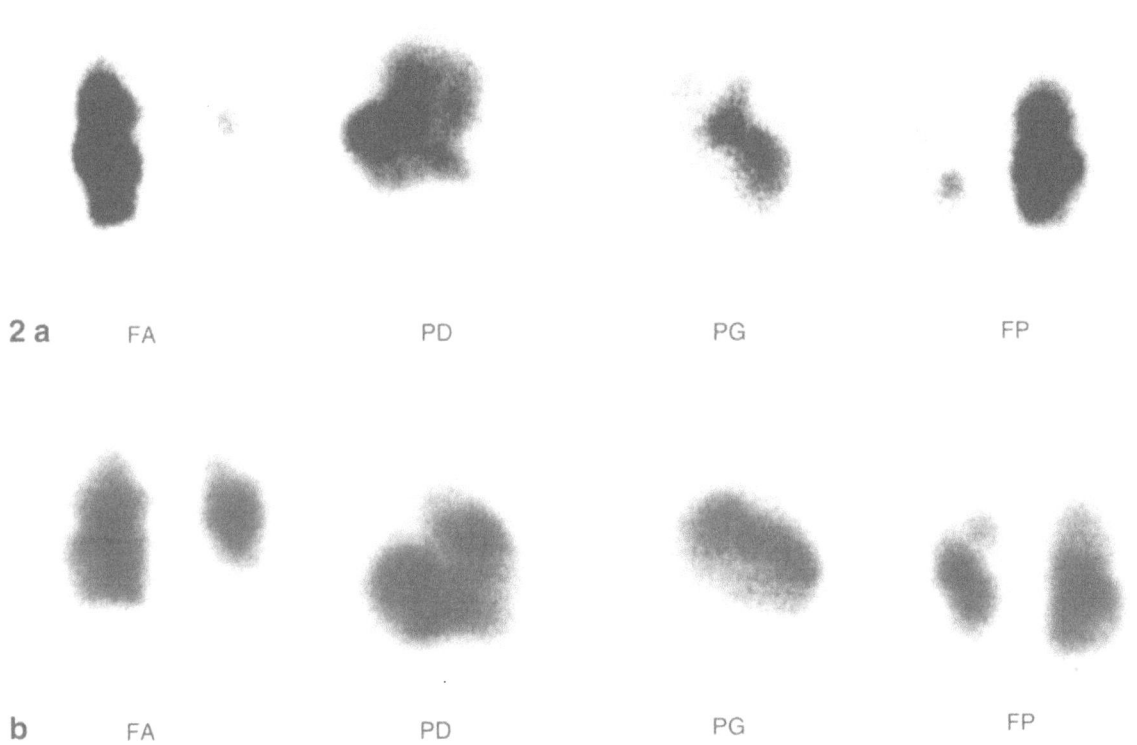

Fig. 2 a, b. Massive pulmonary embolism. **a** Initial perfusion scan showing defect in the whole left lung; **b** follow-up 10 days later. Perfusion is almost normal in the left lung

restrictions of ventilation-perfusion scans in allergic patients with either examination [7].

In conclusion, except in cases with clinical signs suggesting acute major embolism, contra-indications of anti-coagulant therapy, and prior pulmonary embolism without scan control after recovery, pulmonary scintigraphy is the basic technique for the diagnosis of pulmonary embolism. Therefore, organisation is required allowing ventilation-perfusion scintigraphy within a short period. Further investigations to establish pulmonary embolism depend upon scan results on the one hand and local facilities on the other. This point will be discussed in paragraph "Interpretation of pulmonary scintigraphy and diagnostic strategy".

Radionuclide scanning techniques

Pulmonary embolism was the first disease in which the value of lung scanning was demonstrated.

Perfusion scintigraphy

Lung scanning is a simple and effective procedure for the diagnosis of pulmonary embolism. It represents a well established procedure accepted by nuclear medicine physicians. Most centers use approximately 111 MBq (3mCi) of macro-aggregates labeled with technetium-99m. Intravenous injection is usually made in the supine position. To avoid an artefactual nonhomogeneous perfusion, some precautions are necessary. The particles are shaken immediately before injection and the blood must not be allowed to clot within the syringe. The use of multiple projections is critical to proper perfusion imaging. Perfusion lung imaging should include antero-posterior, lateral and oblique views. If properly positioned, the anterior and posterior oblique views provide a good evaluation of perfusion in multiple lung segments [8, 9]. The design of current gamma cameras with gantries suitable for tomographic imaging makes it possible to obtain proper oblique views.

Posterior oblique views improve the definition of lesions in lateral basal segments of the lower lobes. Anterior oblique views provide the best views of the middle lobes. The least helpful of all views are lateral, because of activity superimposition of the lungs. In our laboratory, we usually acquire 400 kcounts in antero-posterior scan. We begin with oblique and lateral views of the less affected lung and acquire 350 kcounts.

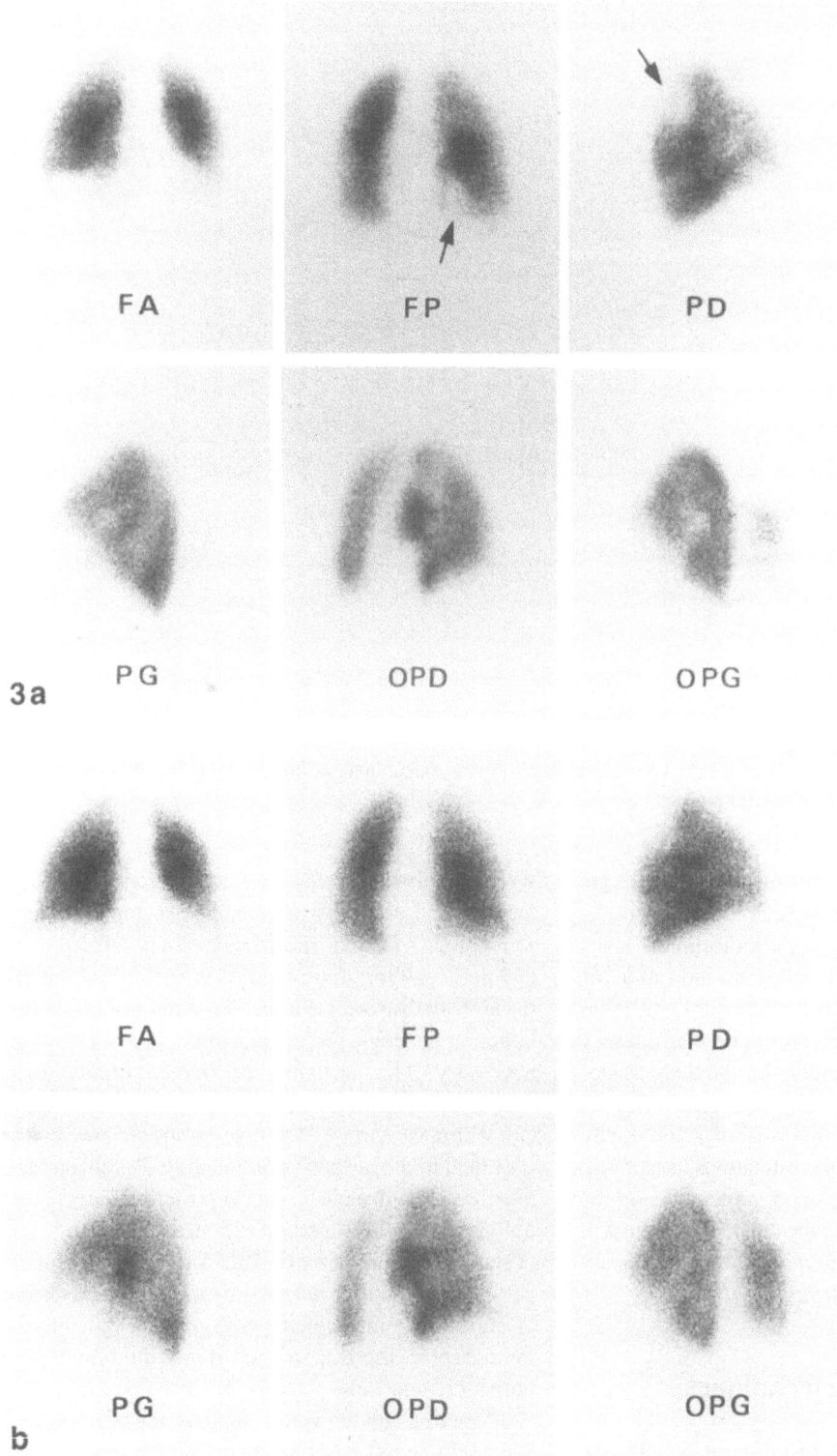

Fig. 3 a, b. Perfusion (99mTc-MAA) **a** and ventilation (99mTc-DTPA) **b** scintigraphy in a patient with right lung emboly. *FA* anterior; *PD* right lateral; *OPD* right posterior oblique; *FP* posterior; *PG* left lateral; *OPG* left posterior oblique. The perfusion scintigraphy shows two defects, in right upper and lower lobes. The ventilation scintigraphy, performed after the perfusion study, vizualizes a filling of these defects. The difference between perfusion and ventilation imaging demonstrates the pulmonary embolism

The contralateral view is obtained for the same time required for the first view.

The interpretation of abnormalities requires a rigorous technique. The scintigraphic data are interpreted in conjunction with a recent good quality chest film. When perfusion defects are obvious, the site and size of defects are established with regard to the bronchopulmonary segmental anatomy and the projection of segments in all views. The size of the defects is usually described in a manner similar to Biello's description [10]. A defect that occupies 75-100% of the segment is segmental. A defect that occupies 25-75% of the segment is subsegmental. The defect is categorized as small if it occupies less than 25% of the segment.

A semi-quantitative evaluation of the lack of perfusion can be accomplished. The usual method consists of using a table representing the normal relative contribution of each lobe of both lungs to perfusion. The normal percentage of lobar vascularization is as follows: right lung-upper lobe = 18%, middle lobe = 12%, lower lobe = 25%; left lung-upper lobe = 13%, lingula = 12%, lower lobe = 20%. The relative hypoperfusion of each lobe is reported. Subsequently, the global perfusion lack is expressed as a percentage of the total pulmonary perfusion.

Pulmonary thrombo-embolism typically creates multiple perfusion defects that are regularly shaped and that extend to the pulmonary surface (fig. 3); the defects are larger at the pleural surface than in the center of the lung. It has been reported that if an area of perfused lung is present between the defect and the pleural surface, the defect is unlikely to be caused by pulmonary embolism [11].

Ventilation scintigraphy

In many cases, ventilation scintigraphy would have to be performed post perfusion. Given the importance of multiple views for the assessment of ventilation perfusion mismatch, it is preferable to use a method that easily permits numerous ventilation views: ideally, the multiple views of perfusion and ventilation would be acquired exactly in the same projection. Several methods for ventilation scanning can be used, each with its advantages and limitations.

Gases

Xenon-133 was the first routine agent used for ventilation imaging and is still currently used [12]. The ventilation study usually begins with a posterior image with an approximately one minute single inhalation of xenon-133. An equilibrium image is obtained. The patient then breathes room air, and the wash-out phase begins. Abnormal areas are seen as regions of decreased activity during the wash-in period and areas of tracer retention during the wash-out phase. In order to provide the best comparison with perfusion imaging, several views should be acquired during the wash-in and wash-out phases. It is frequently difficult to obtain various projections quickly. Xenon-133 scintigraphy is usually performed before the perfusion study to avoid a degradation of the post-perfusion xenon-133 image ($E\gamma$ = 80 kev) by the Compton scattered photons produced by ^{99m}Tc photons ($E\gamma$ = 140 kev). This is a disadvantage of the use of this gas that leads to unnecessary examinations in patients with a normal perfusion scan.

Krypton-81m gas is an almost ideal tracer of ventilation in patients with suspected pulmonary embolism [13]. It can be used post perfusion. It is administered by continuous breathing, so that cooperation is not required and multiple views can easily be obtained. Ventilation abnormalities correspond to areas of decreased activity which can be compared to perfusion abnormalities. However, it is eluted from a very expensive generator and it is not available for routine use.

Aerosols labeled with ^{99m}Tc

Aerosols provide ventilation imaging in multiple views. They use a radiotracer, ^{99m}Tc-DTPA, that is relatively inexpensive. They can be used pre- or post-perfusion. In pre-perfusion study, the nebulizer is filled with about 30 mCi (10^3 MBq). After a perfusion scan, a large amount of radioactivity, up to 80 mCi ($3 \cdot 10^3$ MBq), becomes necessary. A common error consists of performing post perfusion aerosol studies with an insufficient amount of activity. In fact, most of the activity remains in the nebulizer and tubing. The inhaled activity is satisfactory if the pulmonary count rate equals at least three times the pulmonary count rate of the previous perfusion scan.

Regions of hypoventilation correspond to activity defects. Unfortunately, radioaerosols are not gases and in critically ill patients or patients with a severe obstructive disease an excessive central deposition can result in a suboptimal ventilation study. Alderson et al. compared the results of ^{99m}Tc DTPA aerosol with xenon-133 and krypton-81m ventilation scintigraphy: in a small percentage of cases, there was no agreement between aerosol and gas explorations. This was due to an excessive central deposition of aerosols and hot spots; in most patients, the exploration data were concordant.

In spite of these limits, many investigators use ^{99m}Tc DTPA aerosols to search for pulmonary embolism [14] (fig. 3).

Technegas™

A preparation of ^{99m}Tc carbon particles would produce smaller and more uniform particles because the size of particles would result in a much less central deposition. This would have some advantage over the radio-aerosols.

To conclude, the choice of ventilation scintigraphy techniques remains complex. Each nuclear medicine laboratory has to optimize its technique according to its possibilities and the patient population.

Interpretation of pulmonary scintigraphy and diagnostic strategy

The interpretation criteria of pulmonary scan published by the Prospective Investigation of Pulmonary Embolism Diagnosis (PIOPED) investigators [2] are nowadays widely used. Bearing in mind the positive predictive value of lung scan for the diagnosis of pulmonary embolism, they define 5 types of results, i.e. high probability, intermediate probability, low probability, very low probability and normal.

A high probability result corresponds to 3 different scan images highly suggestive of the diagnosis of pulmonary embolism:
– at least 2 large segmental perfusion defects;
– one large segmental perfusion defect (involving more than 75% of considered segments) associated with at least 2 moderate segmental perfusion defects (between 25% and 75% of the considered segments) without equivalent ventilation or chest roentgenogram abnormalities in the same area;
– at least 4 moderate segmental perfusion defects (between 25% and 75% of the considered segments) without equivalent ventilation or chest roentgenogram abnormalities in the same area.

A low probability result corresponds to the following types of scan images:
– no more than 3 large or moderate segmental perfusion defects in one lung region and no more than 4 segmental perfusion defects in the whole lung with matching ventilation defects at least equal in size, and smaller radiographic abnormalities or normal chest X-ray;
– more than 3 small (less than 25% of the considered segments) segmental perfusion defects with normal chest X-ray;
– single moderate segmental perfusion defect (between 25% and 75% of the considered segments) without equivalent ventilation or chest roentgenogram abnormalities in the same area;
– non-segmental perfusion defects
– any perfusion defect with a larger chest X-ray abnormality.

Intermediate probability, also called indeterminate probability, includes cases difficult to categorize as high or low probability.

Very low probability corresponds to cases with no more than 3 small (less than 25% of the considered segments) segmental perfusion defects with normal chest X-ray

Normal corresponds to the absence of perfusion defect.

In order to be analysable in such a manner, pulmonary scintigraphy has to be performed according to the following quality criteria:
– delay between first clinical manifestations and scan less than 48 hours;
– six perfusion images (anterior, posterior, both posterior oblique and anterior oblique views);
– scan performed in the supine position.

In these conditions, a normal ventilation/perfusion scan is considered to eliminate the diagnosis of pulmonary embolism.

In all other cases, diagnosis has to be discussed in terms of the scintigraphic probability defined according to the above criteria, and within the clinical context. Angiogram is the gold standard for the diagnosis of pulmonary embolism. Therefore, it has to be performed in all cases with clinical suspicion of pulmonary embolism (according to clinical examination, chest X-ray, electrocardiography and blood gas analysis) even if the scan exhibits an indeterminate, low or very low probability. In the PIOPED study concerning 931 patients who underwent scintigraphy, of whom 755 also underwent angiogram, this situation was the most frequent. Indeed, only 41% of patients with angiographically proven pulmonary embolism (251 patients) had a high probability scan whereas 42% had an indeterminate scan, 15% had a low probability and 2% a near normal or normal scan.

These results correspond to a ventilation-perfusion scan sensitivity of 41% when considering high probability cases, 82% when considering high and intermediate probability cases, 98% when considering high, intermediate and low probability cases. Specificity was 97% for high probability scans, 52% for high and intermediate probability scans and 10% for high, intermediate and low probability scans. Finally, positive predictive value was 88% in the group of high probability scans, 48% in the group of intermediate scans, and 20% in the group of low probability scans.

Results would be certainly more conflicting if perfusion scans had been performed without ventilation study, especially in patients with cardiopulmonary history. They depend also upon the interpretation criteria which must be precise and clinically relevant as they determine the subsequent strategy of the physician.

References

1. Dalen JE (1991) Clinical diagnosis of acute pulmonary embolism. When should V / Q scan be ordered ? Chest 100 : 1185-1186
2. The PIOPED investigators. Value of the ventilation / perfusion scan in acute pulmonary embolism : results of the prospective investigation of pulmonary embolism diagnosis (PIOPED). JAMA 263 : 2753-2759
3. Conférence de consensus sur la maladie thrombo-embolique veineuse et pulmonaire (1990) J Radiol 71 : 133-145
4. Stein PD, Coleman RE, Gottschalk A et al (1991) Diagnostic utility of ventilation / perfusion lung scans in acute pulmonary embolism is not diminished by pre-existing cardiac or pulmonary disease. Chest 100 : 604-606
5. Lesser BA, Leeper Jr KV, Stein PD et al (1992) The diagnosis of acute pulmonary embolism in patients with chronic obstructive pulmonary disease. Chest 102 : 17-22
6. Peltier P, Planchon B, De Faucal P, Touze MD et al (1988) Embolie pulmonaire et médecine nucléaire J Méd Nucl Biophys 12 : 155-176
7. Conférence de consensus assistance publique (1990) Diagnostic de l'embolie pulmonaire. Concours Med : 112-124
8. Caride VJ, Puri S, Slavin JD et al (1976) The usefulness of posterior oblique views in perfusion lung imaging. Radiol 121 : 669-671
9. Alderson PO, Doppman JL, Diamond SS et al (1978) Ventilation-perfusion lung imaging and selective pulmonary angiography in dogs with experimental pulmonary embolism. J Nucl Med 19 : 164-171
10. Alderson PO, Biello DR, Sachariah KG et al (1981) Scintigraphic detection of pulmonary embolism in patients with obstructive pulmonary disease. Radiology 138 : 661-666
11. Sostman HD, Gottschalk A (1982) The stripe sign : a new sign for diagnosis of non embolic defects on pulmonary perfusion scintigraphy. Radiol 142 : 737-741
12. Alderson PO, Rujanavech N, Secker-Walker RH et al (1976) The role of ^{133}Xe ventilation studies in the scintigraphic detection of pulmonary embolism. Radiology 120 : 633-640
13. Goris ML, Daspit SG (1981) Krypton-81m ventilation scintigraphy for the diagnosis of pulmonary embolism. Clin Nucl Med 6 : 207-212
14. Selby JB, Gallcott F, Gordon L et al (1990) Utility of ^{99m}Tc DTPA aérosol inhalation scans following perfusion lung scans in the diagnosis of pulmonary embolism. Clin Nucl Med 15 : 143-149

Preoperative assessment of pulmonary function

F Baulieu and P Diot

The first successful pneumonectomy was reported in 1933 by Graham and Singer [1]. Since 1955, many studies have focused on morbidity due to respiratory insufficiency after pneumonectomy or even lobectomy. More recently, the development of lung transplantations has increased the necessity for precise pre-operative measurement of pulmonary function. Many techniques have been reported to be useful for such a purpose. Some, such as bronchospirometry, bronchoscopic respiratory gas sampling, temporary unilateral pulmonary arterial occlusion, and intraoperative pulmonary artery pressure measurement [2] have been abandoned now. These techniques are invasive and, in fact, well correlated with non-aggressive tests. Pre-operative measurement of pulmonary function nowadays requires at least spirometry, possibly associated with DLCO and exercise tests. Ventilation and/or perfusion scans complete these basic tests when necessary.

Place of isotopic techniques

Surgical resection is the most effective therapy for most bronchogenic carcinomas. The decision for surgery has to consider resectability and operability [3].

Resectability depends upon the tumor itself and more precisely on the TNM staging. It is defined by the technical possibility for the surgeon to remove the tumor fully. Operability depends upon the patient himself and more precisely on the presumed post-operative pulmonary function. It is defined by the patient's ability to tolerate the consequences of lung resection. Operability is especially critical in patients with lung cancer because their pulmonary function is often compromised by an underlying chronic obstructive pulmonary disease. This problem becomes more and more crucial as age itself no longer contraindicates surgery in physiologically well-preserved patients [4].

A minimum 0.8 liter, or more often 1 liter, expected post operative FEV_1 is usually required to decide pneumonectomy. It has been suggested that reduction of perfusion in the affected lung of less than one third of the total indicates inoperability.

The restrictive effect of pneumonectomy has, as expected, been proven to be well correlated with the pre-operative function of the resected lung. Therefore, it is obviously necessary to appreciate precisely the split function of each lung in patients with pre-operative FEV_1 of less than 2 liters [3].

It is more difficult to predict post-operative pulmonary function after resection of upper lobes or resection of less than 4 pulmonary segments whatever their location.

Post-operative pulmonary function is characterized by two successive stages [5]. Pulmonary function loss is greatest during the first and second post-operative weeks and returns to the predicted value between the fourth and sixth weeks. Although transitory, the acute function loss just after lobectomy has to be taken into consideration, at least in order to be aware of possible early difficulties in some patients.

The functional contribution of the lobe to be resected is difficult to evaluate in view of the anatomic overlapping of different lobes in the same lung. Moreover, there is a gradual increase in volume of the remaining lobes which is significantly greater than the increase in ventilation or perfusion [3]. Therefore,

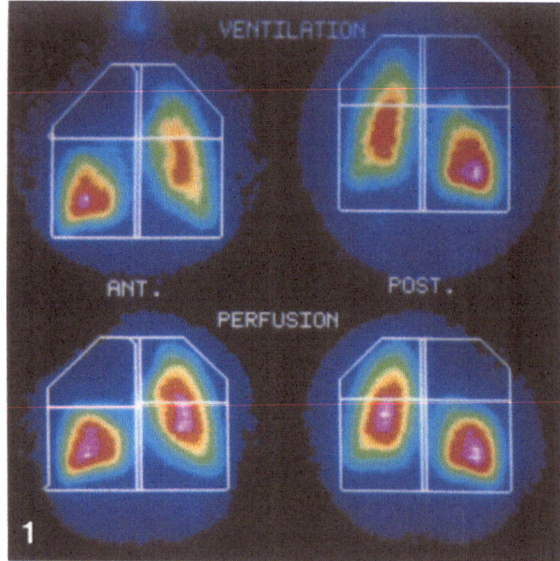

Fig. 1. Ventilation (^{99m}Tc-DTPA) and perfusion (^{99m}Tc-MAA) scintigraphy in a patient with carcinoma in the right upper lobe. The distribution of radio-activity is as follows:

	Right			Left		
	Upper	Lower	Total	Upper	Lower	Total
Ventilation	3%	43%	46%	16%	38%	54%
Perfusion	2%	42%	44%	18%	38%	56%

remaining lobes are hyperinflated and relatively hypoventilated and hypoperfused. The perfusion defect is higher than suggested by endoscopic examinations. Correlations between CT and lung scans remain to be established [6]. Therefore CT belongs to diagnosis and spread study tests whereas ventilation and/or perfusion (V/Q) lung scans serve as functional studies. V/Q scans are not sensitive indicators of mediastinal involvement in patients with lung carcinoma.

The problem of patients with solitary small opacities is easier. In these patients, V/Q scans are either normal or exhibit a defect of equal proportion to the opacity on chest X-ray.

However, isotopic techniques are obviously necessary in patients in whom pulmonary resection can lead to post-operative FEV$_1$ less than 1 liter. In this context, it is important to consider that the pre-operative decision of resection can be modified by anatomic evaluation of the spread of the lesion during surgery. Isotopic techniques are not invasive and are widely available. They should be currently recommended in the pre-operative screening of patients requiring thoracic surgery, especially for lung cancer.

Imaging techniques

Perfusion studies [2, 7]

The technique involves the usual procedure of perfusion scanning, with albumin macroaggregate ^{99m}Tc particles and multiple views.

The interpretation of the scan has to be performed quantitatively to evaluate the pulmonary function. Anterior and posterior views are usually recorded, regions of interest are drawn in both lungs, in anterior and posterior views. The geometric mean of the count is calculated. The contribution of each lung is determined as the percentage of the total perfusion. This test is valuable and easy to perform.

Ventilation studies [3, 6]

The use of ventilation scanning, in conjunction with perfusion, allows a better evaluation of pulmonary function. Numerous ventilation methods are available; gases and aerosols can be used for the pre-operative staging. In most patients with a bronchogenic tumor, a ventilation-perfusion scintigraphy is necessary; therefore, there is no advantage in selecting a tracer that allows ventilation study post-perfusion. The gases (xenon-133, krypton-81m) are specially interesting in patients with broncho-pulmonary disease. Wash-out imaging with xenon-133 would be the most sensitive indicator of ventilatory dysfunction. However, in contrast with radioactive gases, ^{99m}Tc aerosol is inexpensive and easily available in all nuclear medicine departments.

As for perfusion, quantification of ventilation has to be performed. The anterior and posterior views are recorded. Areas of interest are drawn in both lungs in anterior and posterior views. The contribution of each lung is calculated as a percentage of total ventilation.

Protocol example

In our department, the pre-operative scans are performed at one time, using ^{99m}Tc labeled perfusion and ventilation tracers. The investigation begins with ventilation followed by perfusion study. The patient inhales an aerosol of ^{99m}Tc DTPA particles for 3 mn. The nebulizer (Venticis II® CIS Biointernational) is filled with ^{99m}Tc DTPA, about 10^3 MBq (30mCi). The nebulization yield is about 6 to 7%. After the inhalation has been completed, anterior, profiles, oblique and finally posterior views are recorded. After the last acquisition, ^{99m}Tc macroaggregates, 148 MBq (4 mCi), are injected intra-venously, without moving the patient. The residual activity from the previous ventilation study contributes to less than 1/5 of the total activity. The same views are recorded. Anterior and posterior views (400kcounts) are acquired by computer. Each ventilation and perfusion analog image is displayed on film.

The data processing for quantitative analysis is simple to perform. Large, geometric regions of interest (ROI's) are drawn, delineating each lung in anterior and posterior views. The activity of each lung is calculated and expressed as the percentage of activity of both lungs. The calculation is performed on anterior and posterior views for ventilation and perfusion studies. Regional analysis is possible by calculating the activity in sub-regions at the upper or lower part of the lungs or in a region with defective activity. The activity of regional ROI's is expressed as the percentage of the total activity of the lung (fig. 1).

Clinical relevance of lung scans

Requests from surgeons regarding a problem of operability of a patient with lung cancer concerns estimated post-operative ventilation and perfusion.

Major discrepancies between changes in ventilation and perfusion are rare [7]. Nevertheless, it has been shown that some patients with large central tumors have unexpectedly large perfusion defects. This information is obviously of great interest for the surgeon as it reflects not only operability but also in some instances resectability. It is helpful when deciding on an angiogram study. Thus, it appears that ventilation and perfusion scans are both useful and complementary. Ideally, $\dot{V}/\dot{Q}$ scans have to be performed a few days before surgery. Scans must be performed in multiple incidences for both ventilation and perfusion. These conditions allow a precise, quantitated and, if necessary, regional functional evaluation of the lung to be resected.

A qualitative analysis is usually enough for the perfusion study especially bearing in mind that angiogram remains the anatomical gold standard for the surgeon.

The problem of ventilation is very different. Associated with spirometry, ventilation lung scan is the ultimate way to estimate expected post-operative FEV1. Several equations have been suggested for such a purpose.

After pneumonectomy, post operative FEV1 logically corresponds to the following equation: post operative FEV1 = pre operative FEV1 x fraction of contralateral ventilation. It has been shown that a similar result can be obtained using the fraction of contralateral perfusion rather than ventilation.

To estimate pulmonary function loss induced by lobectomy, Khalil Ali [3] proposed the following equation: predicted operative loss = (A/B. Pre f) (Pre F). A is the number of segments to be resected, B the pre-operative number of segments, Pre f the pre-operative regional function as assessed by scan and Pre F the overall pulmonary function as assessed by spirometry. The author suggested the introduction of a correction constant to compensate for deviations due, for example, to heterogeneous contributions of the different segments. Therefore the final equation is: predicted operative loss = (K. A/B. Pre f) (Pre F). K was shown to be approximately 1.26 in short term studies and 0.54 in long term studies. This confirms that early loss in function after lobectomy is greater than expected. On the other hand, the ultimate loss is finally smaller than expected according to the size of anatomical resection. In fact only a tomographic analysis permits precise regional analysis taking into account anatomical superimpositions. Therefore predictions of functional loss after lobectomy are estimations rather than precise evaluations.

References

1. Graham EA, Singer JJ (1933) Successful removal of an entire lung for carcinoma of the bronchus. JAMA 101 : 137

2. Olsen GN, Block AJ, Swenson EW et al (1975) Pulmonary function evaluation of the lung resection candidate : a prospective study. Am Rev Respir Dis 111 : 379-387

3. Khalil Ali M, Mountain CF, Ewer MS et al (1980) Predicting loss of pulmonary function after pulmonary resection for bronchogenic carcinoma. Chest 77 : 337-342

4. Boysen PG, Harris JO, Block AJ et al (1981) Prospective evaluation for pneumonectomy using perfusion scanning. Follow-up beyond one year. Chest 80 : 163-66

5. Pelletier C, Lapointe L, Le Blanc P (1990) Effects of lung resection on pulmonary function and exercise capacity. Thorax 45 : 497-502

6. Lipscomb DJ, Pride NB (1977) Ventilation and perfusion scans in the preoperative assessment of bronchial carcinoma. Thorax 32 : 720-725

7. Boysen PG, Block AJ, Olsen GN et al (1977) Prospective evaluation for pneumonectomy using the ^{99m}Tc Quantitative perfusion lung scan. Chest 72 : 422-425

Diffuse interstitial lung diseases

P Diot, E Lemarié, A Le Pape, P Peltier and N Caillat-Vigneron

Current concepts

Diffuse interstitial lung diseases (ILD) constitute a heterogenous group of processes which have in common reticular or nodular, reticulonodular or linear patterns on chest roentgenogram. They are characterized by a diffuse infiltration of alveolar walls by inflammatory or malignant cells, connective tissue or fluid. About 100 entities have been ascribed to diffuse interstitial lung disease. The aim of the clinician is to confirm the diagnosis of ILD, to elicit an entity from history, symptoms, physical examination, chest roentgenogram, pulmonary function and laboratory data in order to plan treatment. Therefore, the pattern may include malignant, infectious, and cardiac diseases with roentgenographic reticulo-nodular patterns, i.e lymphangitic carcinomatosis, alveolar cell carcinoma, miliary tuberculosis, infection in immunosuppressed patients, and congestion of the lungs secondary to congestive heart failure. In fact, the term ILD usually excludes this heterogenous group of diseases and is focused on inflammatory processes in which the common outcome is dominated by fibrotic lung disorder. They are also commonly called pulmonary fibrosis and will be developed in this chapter.

Thus defined, ILD constitute a group of chronic diseases of different causes in which the final common outcome is the destruction of the normal structure of alveoli, terminal bronchioles and small pulmonary blood vessels. Until recently, these lung disorders were considered to be "interstitial", reflecting the concept that the fibrosis was limited to the interstitium of the alveolar walls. It is now established that the fibrotic process is intra-alveolar as well as interstitial. Although clinical and functional features of most of these diseases are similar, some particular aspects including characteristic appearance on computed tomography (CT) and laboratory data are useful for diagnosis. Tissue sampling is often required in order to define the process precisely and to choose adequate treatment [1].

Pathogenesis: alveolitis and fibrosis

Independent of their origin, the first step is an inflammation of the lower respiratory tract called "alveolitis". Injury causes the destruction of type I cells and also causes breaks in the basement membrane. There is edema in the alveolar airspace and infiltration of the interstitial content by inflammatory cells. The second step is a repair process. The damaged type I cells are replaced by proliferating type II cells. Mesenchymal cells proliferate with deposition of connective tissue. Interstitial contents move into the alveolar airspace, causing intra-alveolar fibrosis. The alveolar walls are thickened. There is considerable disturbance in the architecture often concerning respiratory bronchioles [1].

Disorders such as sarcoidosis, histiocytosis X or idiopathic pulmonary fibrosis (IPF) are characterized by different types of inflammation, dominated by alveolar macrophages (AM), neutrophils, lympho-cytes and/or eosinophils. Among these disorders, IPF is a good example of a process consistent with the concept that it is inflammation that causes the fibrosis (fig. 1). Alveolitis is dominated by AM and neutrophils that promote the subsequent injury and fibrosis.

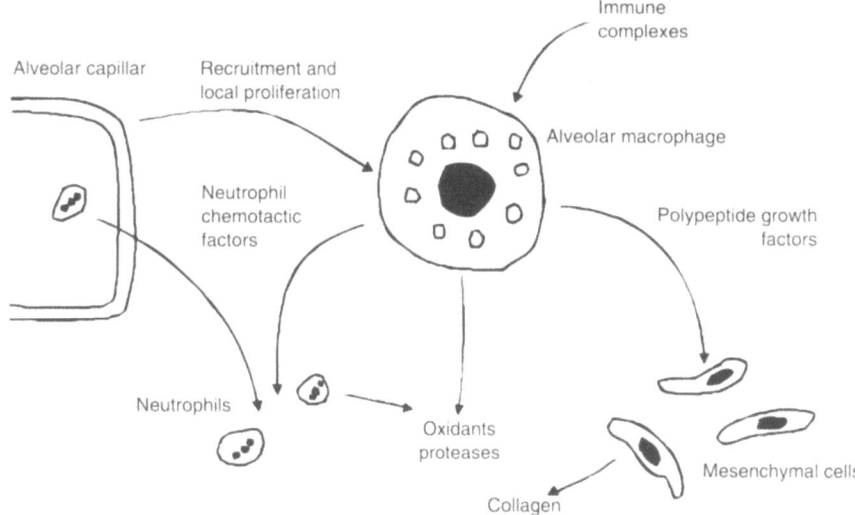

Fig 1. Mechanisms of injury and biologic processes associated with idiopathic pulmonary fibrosis

Eosinophils and basophils/mast cells also contribute to the injury. AM are the centre of inflammation. Monocytes are attracted to the lungs and proliferate locally. AM release chemoattractants for neutrophils and oxydants which play a direct role in parenchymal injury. They also release growth signals for mesenchymal cells. Neutrophils accumulate in the lung, and release oxydants and proteases such as collagenase and neutrophil elastase. Eosinophils, which are very few in number in the healthy lung, also accumulate in IPF lungs and release oxydants, collagenase and other agents such as major basic protein. Lung T cells direct B cells to produce immunoglobulins. Mesenchymal cells, which are in increased numbers in the interstitium, synthesize type I collagen and other matrix components. Alveolar walls are thickened with collagen fibers [2].

Diffuse interstitial lung disease from the perspective of the clinician [1]

The most common diffuse interstitial lung diseases are listed in table 1. In approximately two-thirds of cases, there is a known etiology: hypersensitivity pneumonitis, inorganic pneumoconioses and drug induced pulmonary diseases. In one-third of cases, the etiology is immunologic (collagen diseases) or unknown: sarcoidosis, idiopathic pulmonary fibrosis, lymphangioleiomyomatosis, histiocytosis X and neurofibromatosis.

The history of the disease is usually progressive dyspnea with chronic cough. Fever is unusual except for patients with infection. Drug exposure such as immunosuppressants (glucocorticoids and cytotoxic agents) or other drugs administered for long periods (nitrofurantoin, gold and amiodarone), environmental exposure (silica, asbestos and organic dusts), previous history of rheumatoid arthritis or other collagen diseases should alert the attention of the clinician. The typical breathing pattern is tachypnea either at rest or with exercise. In contrast, patients with sarcoidosis are frequently asymptomatic. Auscultation reveals classic "velcro" rales at the bases. Digital clubbing is observed in the late stages of histiocytosis X. Cutaneous lesions can be seen in patients with sarcoidosis, histiocytosis X and collagen diseases.

Chest roentgenogram shows reticulonodular infiltrates involving all lobes of both lungs. There may be zonal predominance. High resolution computerized tomography (HRCT) appears to be particularly valuable in elucidating characteristic distributions of disease which suggest specific entities. Accentuation of the upper and middle zones is characteristic of sarcoidosis, histiocytosis X (fig. 2) or silicosis whereas involvement of the lower zones predominates in asbestosis and scleroderma. In IPF the chest X-ray reveals diffuse reticulonodular infiltrates, also prominent at the bases. Bilateral hilar lymphadenopathy associated with lung infiltrates is characteristic of sarcoidosis. Pleural calcifications may be associated with asbestosis. HRCT scan is essential to assess the extent of the fibrotic process and the alveolar infiltration.

Pulmonary function tests show a decrease in lung volumes and impairment of carbon monoxyde diffusing capacity (DLCO). The restrictive pattern is

Table 1. Diffuse interstitial lung disease: chief entities

	Entity	History	Chest roentgenogram characteristics	Blood investigations	Bronchoalveolar lavage
ILD with known etiology	Hypersensitivity pneumonitis (farmer's lung, pigeon breeder)	Environmental exposure to organic dusts		Precipitating antibodies	Increased lymphocytes
	Pneumoconiosis (asbestos, silica, beryllium)	Environmental exposure to inorganic dusts	Pleural calcification: asbestosis Hilar "eggshell": silicosis Hilar adenopathy: berylliosis		Increased neutrophils: asbestosis Increased lymphocytes: berylliosis
	Drug-induced pulmonary disease	Drug exposure: cytotoxic agents, nitrofurantoin, gold, amiodarone, etc.		Immunologic tests	Increased lymphocytes
ILD with unknown etiology	Collagen disease	Collagen disease: rheumatoid arthritis, scleroderma, Dermatomyositis Sjogren syndrome	Prominent in lung bases Pleural effusion (rheumatoid arthritis)	Rheumatoid factor Antinuclear antibodies and other autoantibodies	
	Histiocytosis X		Pneumothorax, Honeycombing		X bodies in macrophages
	Sarcoidosis		Hilar adenopathy Upper and mid zone predominance	Angiotensin-converting enzyme activity, Increased neopterin Hypercalcemia, Hypercalcuria	Increased lymphocytes
	Neurofibromatosis		Bullae		
	Lymphangioleio-myomatosis	Pleural effusion	Pneumothorax		
	Idiopathic pulmonary fibrosis	Prominent in lung bases	Honeycombing		Increased neutrophils

usually seen in the absence of obstruction of the airways. Initially, arterial blood gas tests reveal a fall in resting PaO_2 which decreases with exercise. Ventilation-perfusion mismatching is present, reflecting the physiologic process that produces hypoxemia. The degree of abnormalities in pulmonary function tests and blood gas levels is a function of the severity of the disease.

Bronchoalveolar lavage (BAL) is an important tool in the diagnosis of diffuse interstitial lung diseases. Increased lymphocytes in BAL are common in sarcoidosis. In hypersensivity pneumonitis, increased lymphocytosis, greater than that in sarcoidosis, is

encountered. The ratio of thymus-dependent helper cells to thymus-dependent suppressor cells is greater than in sarcoidosis whereas this ratio is reversed in hypersensitivity pneumonitis. An increased percentage of neutrophils in BAL is characteristic in IPF and other interstitial lung diseases such as sarcoidosis at their end fibrotic stage. Histiocytosis can be diagnosed on finding X bodies in the macrophages from BAL.

Some blood investigations may be helpful in diagnosis (table 1). In sarcoidosis, elevated levels of serum angiotensin-converting enzyme activity (SACE) are found in approximately 80% of patients

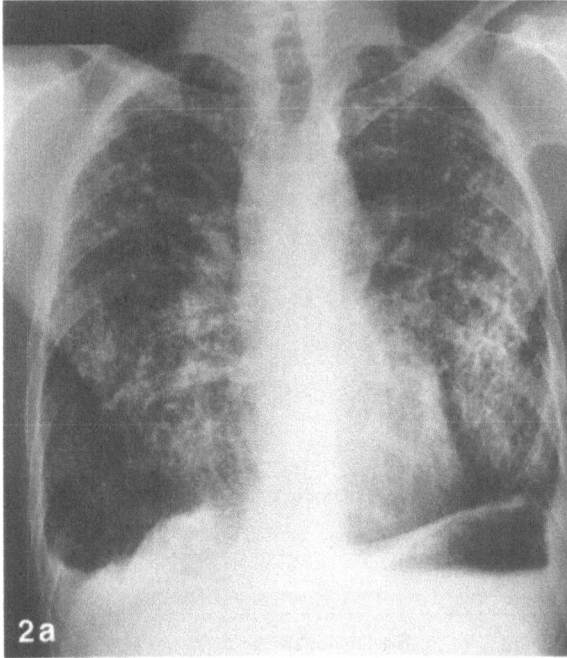

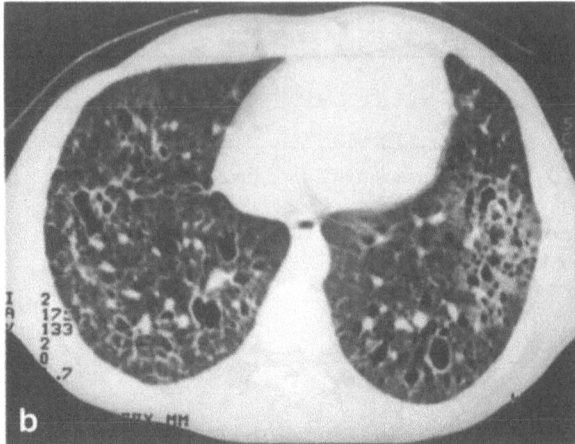

Fig 2 a, b. Histiocytosis X. **a** Posteroanterior roentgenogram reveals extensive bilateral pulmonary disease with maximum involvement in the mid-lung zones; **b** high resolution CT scan through the base of both lungs reveals a multitude of cystic spaces

with sarcoidosis. In hypersensitivity pneumonitis, appropriate serologic tests should be made according to history of exposure. Antinuclear antibodies and other autoantibodies are essential in collagen diseases. Tissue sampling is always necessary to assess the diagnosis of diffuse interstitial lung disease. The technique of choice may differ according to clinical, radiological and laboratory data: mediastinoscopy, transbronchial lung biopsy, open lung biopsy.

Markers of activity

Although fibrosis is the final stage of the disease, its degree varies among patients and is associated with a certain degree of inflammation. Patients with predominently cellular histopathology have the most favorable prognosis (2). In practice, repeated biopsy specimens cannot be sampled. Noninvasive markers of activity are required to determine the stage of the disease and the degree of inflammation present and to assess the impact of therapy (2).

Physiologic markers include increased lung elastic recoil, reduced lung volumes, decreased DLCO and hypoxemia that are generally correlated with lung fibrosis in IPF patients. In contrast, pulmonary function tests tend to correlate poorly with chest roentgenogram and histologic samples in pulmonary sarcoidosis. The major usefulness of pulmonary function tests in sarcoidosis patients appears to be for

following the course of the disease using sequential measurements.

Bronchoalveolar lavage is an important tool to understand inflammatory and immune processes involved in diffuse interstitial lung diseases. Patterns of inflammation such as the percentage of lymphocytes in BAL have not been proved to be correlated with disease activity in sarcoidosis. In IPF, the presence of ≥ 5% neutrophils in BAL fluid is indicative of clinical progression but it does not appear to provide a quantitative marker of disease activity. However, an increased number of BAL fluid lymphocytes is thought to be predictive of a favorable response to corticoid therapy.

Gallium-67 lung scans are frequently abnormal in patients with pulmonary sarcoidosis and other ILD. In sarcoidosis, a positive gallium scan is correlated with the response to therapy in some studies but not in others. Nevertheless, a negative scan appears to be useful information indicating that the patient does not require therapy. In ILD other than sarcoidosis, the usefulness of gallium scan in routine evaluation is not clearly defined.

Untreated sarcoidosis patients with active clinical disease tend to have greater elevations of SACE. This test is probably valuable to evaluate the total body burden of the disease and to determine the need for therapy, especially for patients with extrapulmonary manifestations.

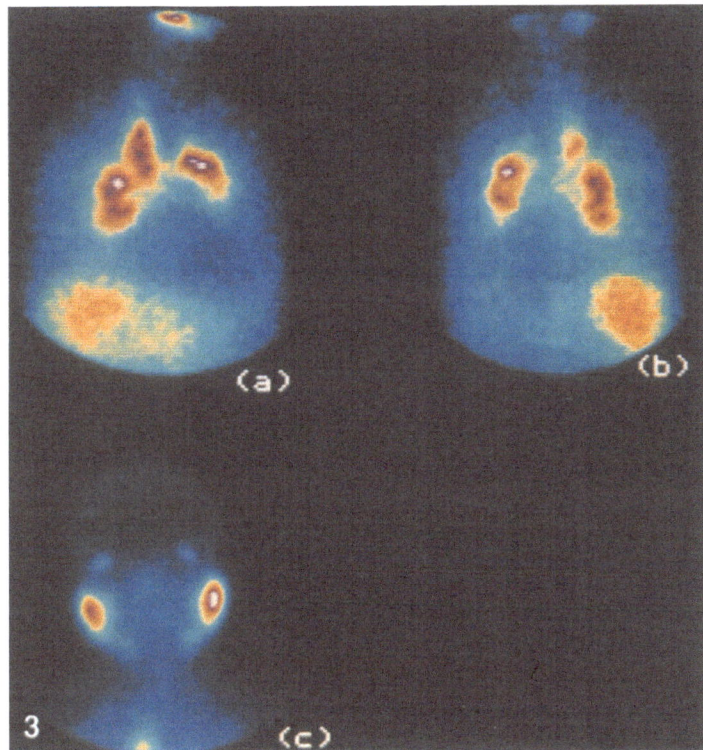

Fig. 3. Gallium-67 imaging of sarcoidosis (stage 1). Anterior *(a)* and posterior *(b)* views of the chest, anterior view of the head *(c):* a combination of the "lambda" and "panda" images

Radionuclide scanning techniques

Gallium-67 scanning

Mechanisms of gallium-67 accumulation in inflammatory lesions

Chronic inflammation is characterized by a proliferative response of tissue to injury, with a predominantly mononuclear cell infiltration (macrophages, lymphocytes and plasma cells). This proliferation is chiefly fibroblastic and vascular. Transferrin-gallium-67 complex is delivered to the inflammatory lesions through capillaries with increased permeability [3], but no report has shown whether or not the uptake of gallium-67 into the inflammatory tissue was consistent with the uptake of transferrin [4]. Lactoferrin discharged by the leukocytes on the site of inflammation tends to remain localized on receptor sites in tissue macrophages. Gallium-67 may be retained by binding to lactoferrin [5].

Pulmonary sarcoidosis

Gallium-67 scintigraphy is widely used as an aid in diagnosis and in evaluation of the activity of the disease. Gallium-67 uptake depends on the extent of the granulomatous inflammation in involved organs and has proved to be more sensitive than chest radiographs [6]. The mechanism of uptake in sarcoid lesions seems to be related to activated T- and B-lymphocytes and macrophages as opposed to epithelioid cells which produce an excess of angiotensin-converting enzyme.

Gallium uptake is not specific of sarcoidosis. However, intense accumulation in bilateral, symmetrical hilar lymphadenopathy and salivary glands ("lambda" sign and "panda" appearance) (stage 1), (fig. 3) often associated with parenchymal infiltration, mainly posterior (stage 2) (fig. 4), is highly suggestive of sarcoidosis [7] This specific anatomic lymph node distribution correlates well with the normal lymph node group distribution in man. Nevertheless, diagnosis must be based primarily on histological findings and the detection of pulmonary inflammation can guide transbronchial biopsy. Accumulation in the spleen (fig. 5), enlarged liver, skin sarcoids (fig. 6), skeletal muscle, lacrimal glands, finger bones and sometimes the myocardium (fig. 7), together with other activity markers, enhance specificity.

Serum angiotensin-converting enzyme (SACE) level and bronchoalveolar lavage (BAL) have also been widely used to assess disease activity. Comparing SACE activity to gallium-67 in terms of sensitivity and

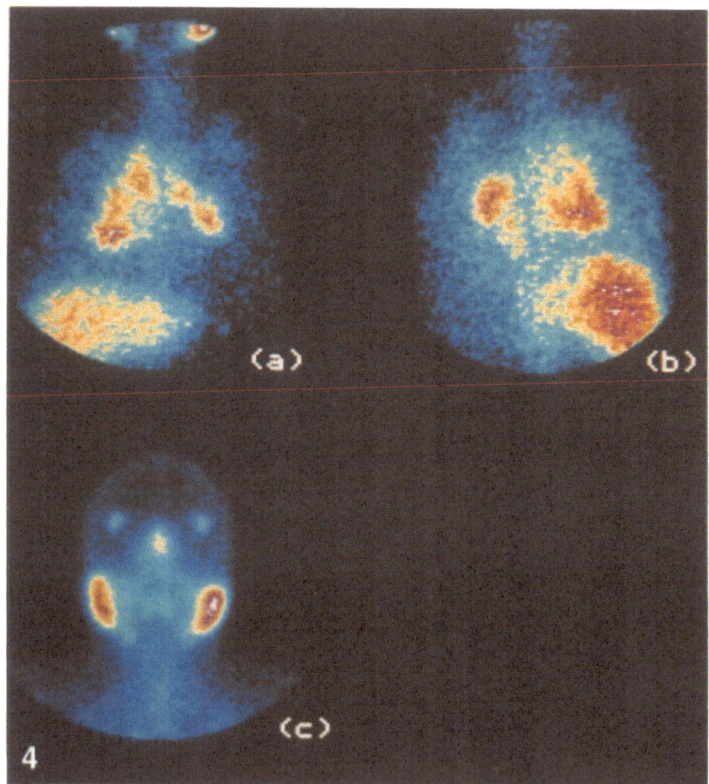

Fig. 4. Gallium-67 imaging of sarcoidosis (stage 2). Anterior *(a)* and posterior *(b)* views of the chest, anterior view of the head *(c)*: bilateral hilar adenopathy with pulmonary involvement and "panda" appearance

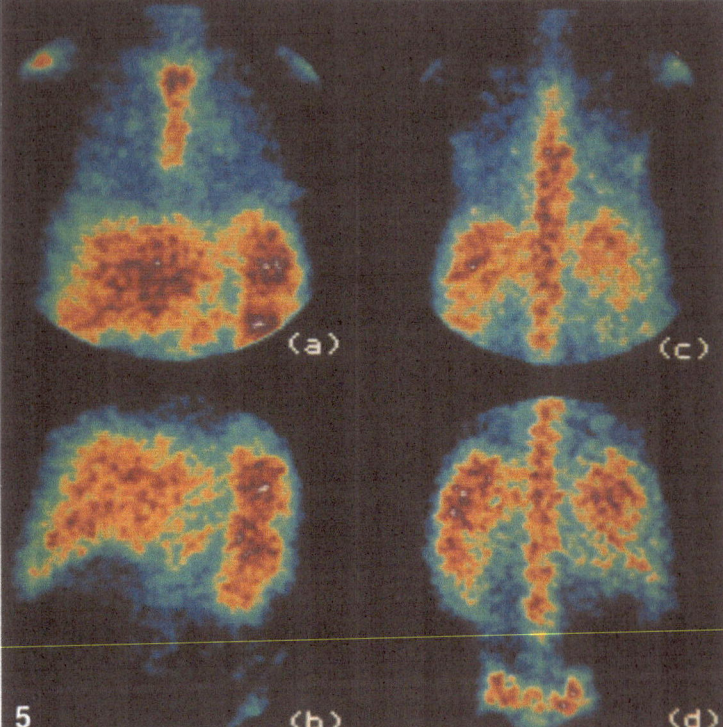

Fig. 5. Hepatosplenic and bone marrow uptake of gallium-67 in the course of organomegaly related to sarcoidosis. Anterior *(a)* and posterior *(c)* views of the chest, anterior *(b)* and posterior *(d)* views of the abdomen

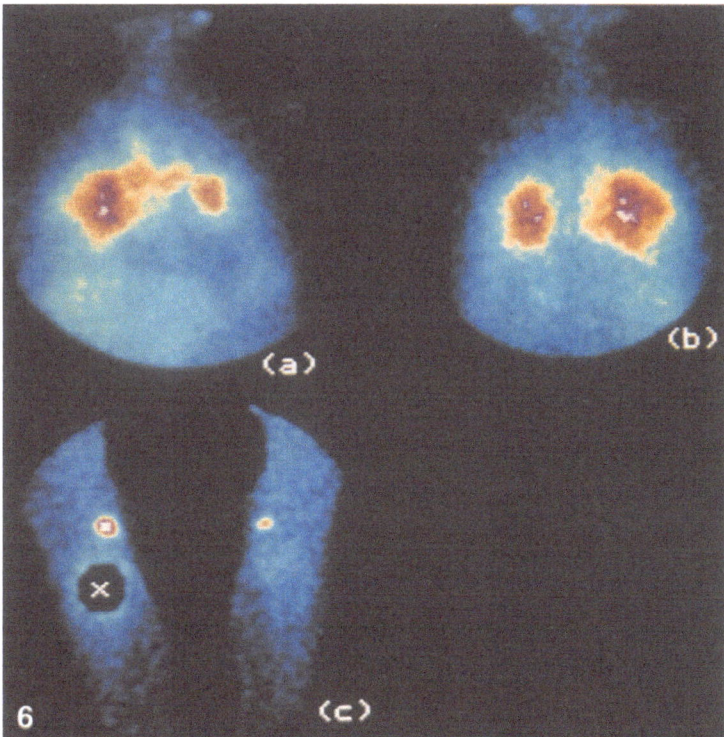

Fig. 6. Gallium-67 imaging of sarcoidosis. Prominent pulmonary uptake on anterior *(a)* and posterior *(b)* views of the chest. bilateral uptake of gallium-67 in skin sarcoids of the arms *(x* site of injection)

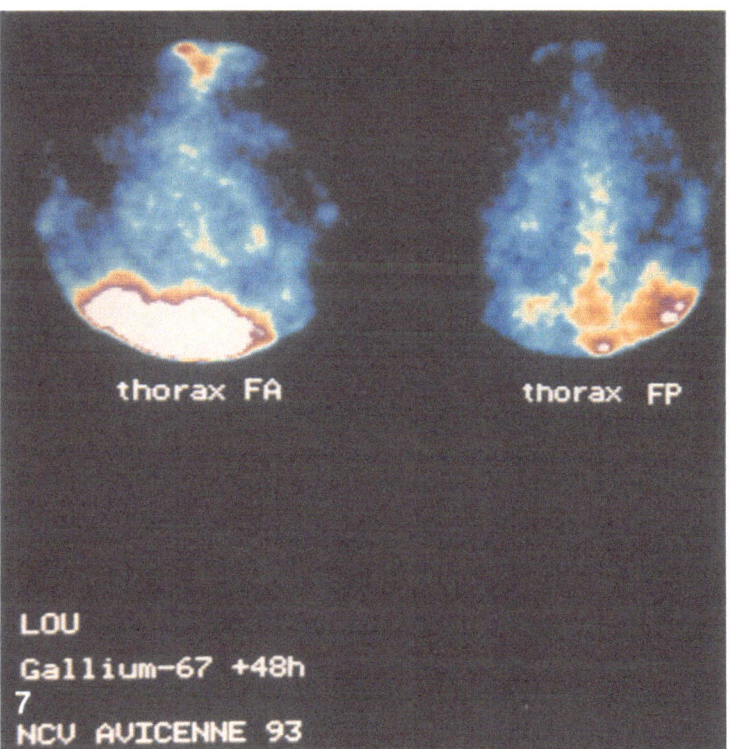

Fig. 7. Gallium-67 imaging of sarcoidosis. Anterior *(FA)* and posterior *(FP)* views of the chest: myocardial uptake

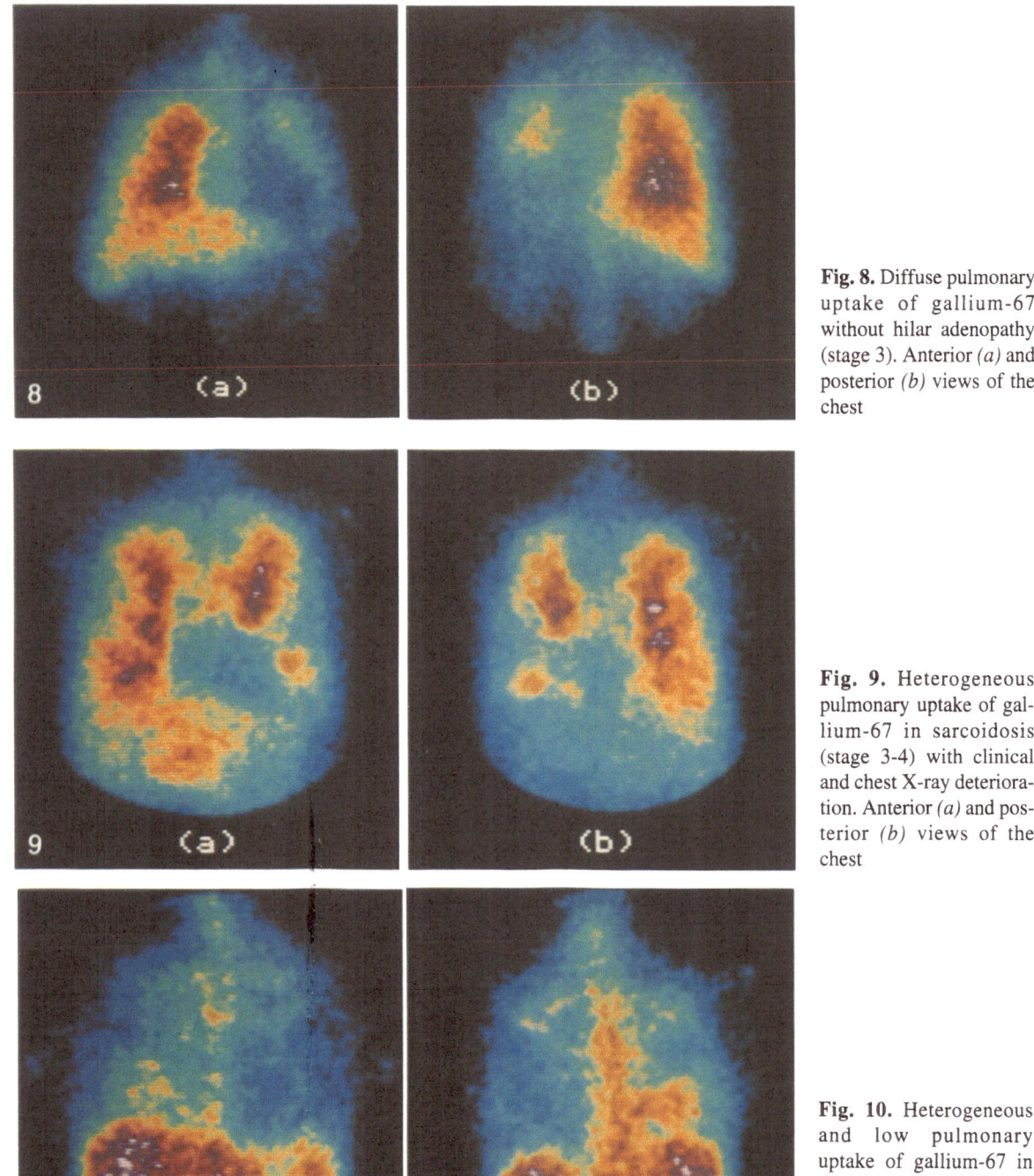

Fig. 8. Diffuse pulmonary uptake of gallium-67 without hilar adenopathy (stage 3). Anterior (a) and posterior (b) views of the chest

Fig. 9. Heterogeneous pulmonary uptake of gallium-67 in sarcoidosis (stage 3-4) with clinical and chest X-ray deterioration. Anterior (a) and posterior (b) views of the chest

Fig. 10. Heterogeneous and low pulmonary uptake of gallium-67 in sarcoidosis with irreversible fibrotic changes in the pulmonary interstitium. Anterior (a) and posterior (b) views of the chest

specificity, gallium-67 proved to be more sensitive and most of the authors did not find any correlation between the SACE level and the response to therapy [8-11]. SACE has been identified in the endothelial cells of the

granuloma and this may explain the weak correlation found between SACE and alveolitis. BAL samples only a portion of the lung (lingula or right lower lobe) and cannot assess whole lung inflammation. For this

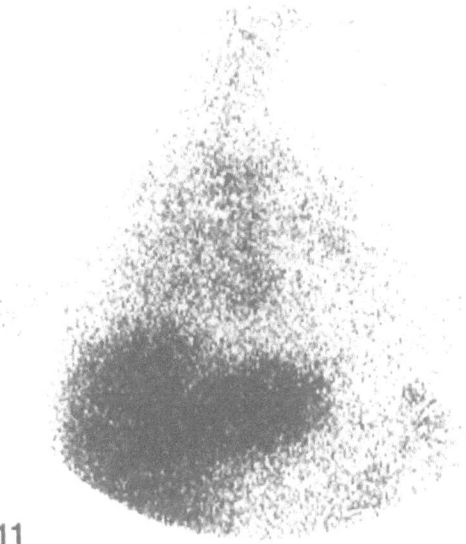

Fig. 11. Pulmonary uptake of gallium-67 in the lesions of Histiocytosis X mainly localized in the right upper lobe of the lungs (anterior view)

11

reason, there is a poor correlation between the results of lymphocyte count in BAL fluid and the activity of the whole lungs evaluated with gallium-67 scintigraphy [12]. Furthermore, large variations are found in the lymphocyte count in BAL fluid from different portions of the lung. The abnormalities in BAL fluid are also related to the pattern of lymphocyte subpopulations; they are almost all T-lymphocytes with a prominent amount of activated T-lymphocytes and frequent modifications of the T4-T8 ratio [13]. The number and status of transferrin membrane receptors are key parameters of cell activation. Gallium-67 regional activity may be closely related to this cell status. These activity markers are thus complementary rather than concordant and each of them should be interpreted in the light of its advantages and limitations regarding the assessment of physiopathological processes in the course of the disease.

Dramatic improvement in pulmonary function can be obtained in the active stage with corticosteroids but the advantages of routine use of steroids have never been demonstrated. Chest radiographs and pulmonary function tests are not predictive of a patient's clinical course as they cannot distinguish between active inflammation and irreversible fibrosis [14]. When used selectively, gallium-67 scintigraphy is valuable for monitoring therapy, showing improvement or resolution of areas of abnormal uptake in the absence of radiographic changes (figs. 8-10).

Some authors emphasize the use of computerized quantification to improve the value of gallium-67 activity in the lungs [10, 13, 15]. Pulmonary sarcoid lesions are usually distributed heterogeneously and no

distinction can easily be made between an active node and a diffuse spread of equal intensity. Furthermore, liver uptake is still often proposed as a reference for gallium uptake in spite of major criticisms. Physiological hepatic uptake varies greatly from one patient to another with the level of transferrin and lactoferrin in the blood and different disorders including sarcoidosis itself (see fig. 5) or hepatitis preclude its use for quantification [16]. Different methods have been proposed using soft tissue background (on the shoulders or on the posterior abdomen) or the injected dose as a reference

Histiocytosis X

Histiocytosis X or pulmonary eosinophilic granuloma, are not true granulomas and the presence of eosinophils is not constant. This disorder is easy to confuse with sarcoidosis, although the rarity of hilar adenopathy favors histiocytosis X. The disease is characterized by the accumulation of atypical histiocytes in the form of parenchymal nodules, and remains confined to the lung in the vast majority of adult patients.

Gallium-67 scintigraphy findings in pulmonary histiocytosis X are of lower activity than those of sarcoid lesions, without the patchy intense uptake with mediastinal and hilar involvement in sarcoidosis. Gallium-67 uptake is fairly often diffuse and heterogeneous, involving the whole lung with relative sparing of the lung bases (fig. 11).

Spontaneous remissions are common and, in the case of persistance of active disease, gallium-67 lung-scanning may be of value in follow-up studies of

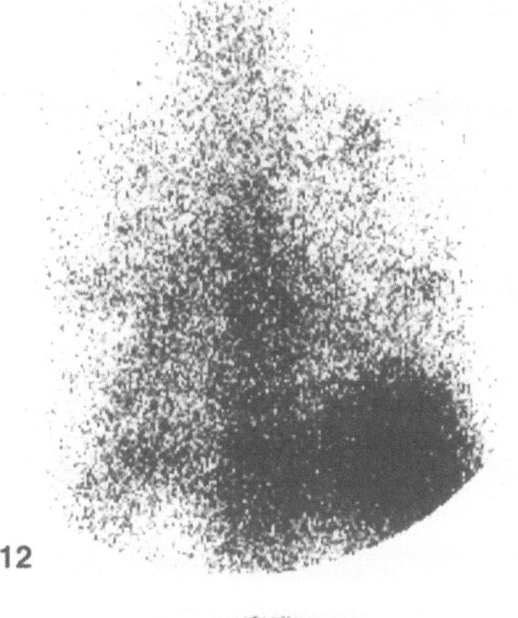

12

Fig. 12. Chronic eosinophilic pneumonia: heterogeneous lung uptake of gallium-67 showing peripheral nodules in the right lung (posterior view)

Fig. 13 a, b. Diffuse bilateral gallium-67 uptake at the early phase of idiopathic pulmonary fibrosis. **a** Anterior and **b** posterior views of the chest. The proximal and posterobasal intensification of activity is obvious

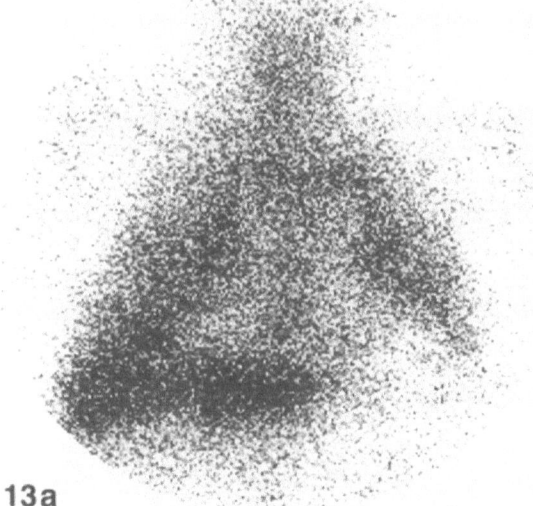

13a

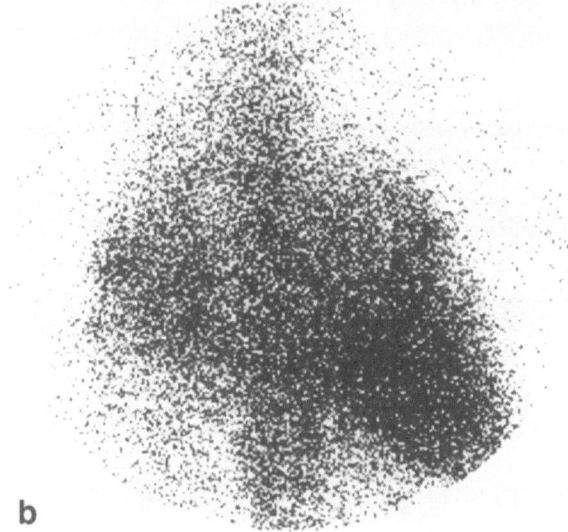

b

patients. Bone involvement, typically affecting children, is also delineated on gallium-67 scintigraphy.

Wegener's granulomatosis

Wegener's granulomatosis is a necrotizing vasculitis classically involving the lung, the upper respiratory tract and the kidneys. Lung involvement usually consists of nodular lesions of varying size. Cavitation within a large nodule is a frequent occurrence. Bacterial colonization of any localisation can be observed, enhancing gallium-67 uptake within the cavity and on the margin of the nodules.

Pulmonary infiltrates with eosinophilia

Infiltration of the pulmonary interstitium with eosinophils has been described in many diverse disorders. This disease is an often recurrent, symptomatic chronic eosinophilic pneumonia. It refers to the presence of parenchymal opacities with peripheral eosinophilia. The symptoms are severe, steroid responsive but steroid dependant and relapse may occur once treatment is discontinued. Gallium-67 scintigraphy can be used to follow the course of the disease and the response to therapy (fig. 12).

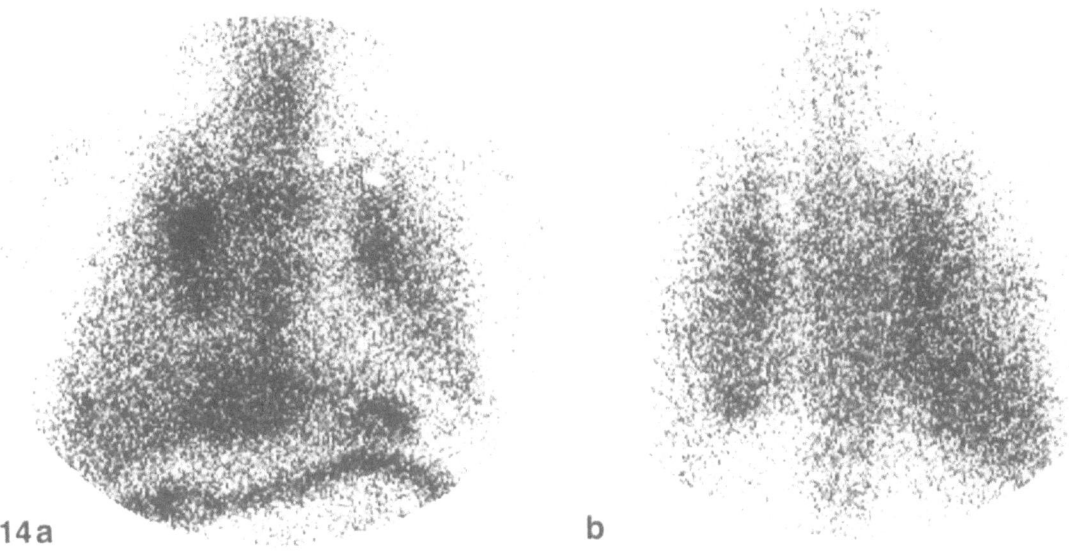

Fig. 14 a, b. Late active pulmonary fibrosis: intense bilateral activity of Gallium-67 uptake in the central area of the lung showing a characteristic pattern of advanced idiopathic pulmonary fibrosis. **a** Anterior and **b** posterior views of the chest

Idiopathic pulmonary fibrosis or usual interstitial pneumonia (UIP)

The inflammatory phase of the disease may precede and probably induce the fibrotic state. Several authors found a close correlation with the degree of interstitial and alveolar cellularity on biopsy and with neutrophil count in BAL fluid. Intensity of gallium uptake in the lungs of patients with UIP is probably associated with an acute inflammatory phase and therapeutic improvement can be expected. Chest X-ray demonstrates a reticular or reticulonodular pattern in the case of established interstitial fibrosis but has yielded disappointing results for asymptomatic patients or staging of disease activity early in the course of therapy. High values of regional pulmonary DTPA-technetium-99m clearance rate together with abnormal gallium-67 lung uptake (fig. 13) can help to differentiate UIP from scleroderma in the early phase of these diseases. The DTPA clearance rate is significantly higher in UIP than in scleroderma and often the distribution of gallium-67 into the lung parenchyma is different (figs. 13-16).

Interstitial lung disease associated with connective tissue diseases

Connective tissue diseases are often referred to as collagen vascular disorders and include Systemic Lupus Erythematosus (SLE), Progressive Systemic Sclerosis (PSS), Polymyositis-Dermatomyositis (PDM), Sjögren's Syndrome (SS), and Rheumatoid

Arthritis (RA). The symptoms and signs of these disorders tend to be variable and overlapping.

The value of scintigraphic imaging is mainly in the investigation of the manifestations of these diseases in the axial interstitium (peribronchovascular connective tissue sheaths) and lung parenchyma. In addition to the identification of pulmonary interstitial fibrosis (UIP), the connective tissue diseases have contributed to the identification of other pulmonary syndromes: lymphocytic interstitial pneumonitis (LIP), alveolar hemorrhage (AH), and bronchiolitis obliterans (BO).

Interstitial Fibrosis is probably the end result of repeated episodes of acute alveolitis or diffuse alveolar damage [17]. It is characterized by the accumulation of mesenchymal cells and their extracellular matrix throughout the pulmonary parenchyma. The chest X-ray findings may remain normal for a long time [18] and, in order to avoid open-chest lung biopsy, additional investigations are indicated to confirm the diagnosis and to evaluate the prognosis: pulmonary function tests, bronchoalveolar lavage, chest CT-scan, and gallium-67 scintigraphy.

Bronchoalveolar lavage [19, 20] cannot depict specific abnormalities in UIP and usually reveals abnormally high numbers of polymorphonuclear neutrophils and lymphocytes (CD8 rather than CD4).

High resolution computed tomography [21, 22] most often reveals peripherally distributed reticular, fine-meshed lesions, associated with "ground glass" hyperdense areas and bronchiectasis caused by traction.

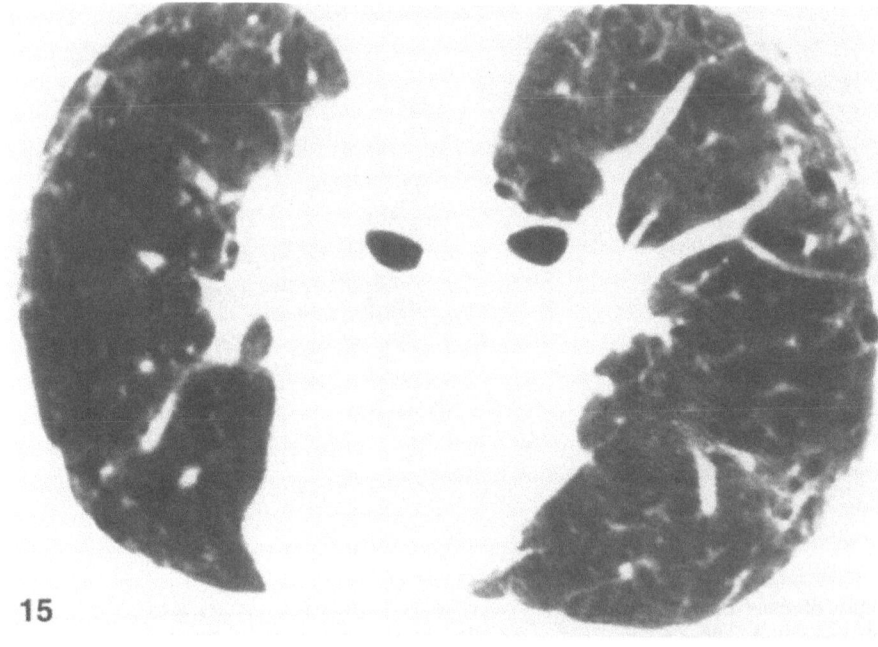

Fig. 15. alveolitis intermingled with fibrosis in scleroderma: the CT-scan demonstrates basal and peripheral honeycombing, groundglass opacities, small cysts with small linear shadows and thickening of alveolar walls

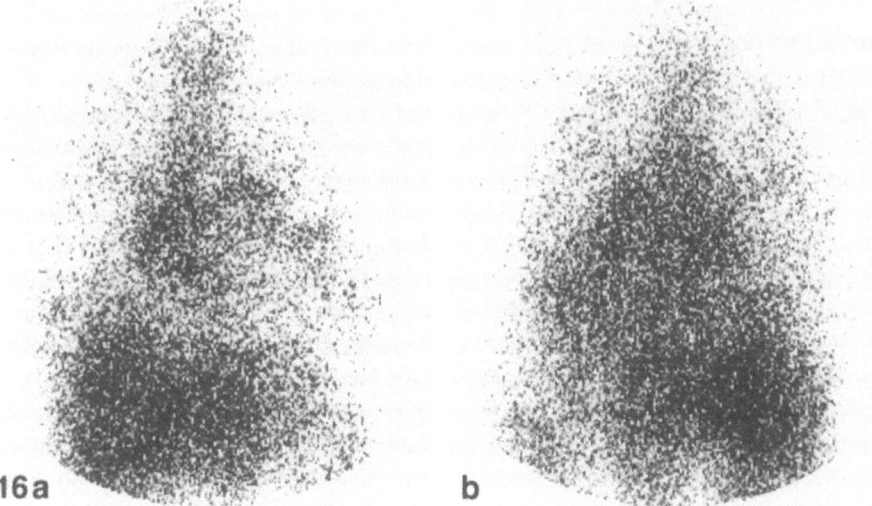

Fig. 16 a, b. Gallium-67 scintigraphy of the same patient with scleroderma shows the typical triangular-shaped posterior distribution of active lesions. **a** Anterior and **b** posterior views of the chest

Areas with a reticular pattern are intermingled with areas of normal lung and the distribution of the disease is predominantly subpleural and dorsal [23]. Cystic spaces are often observed until, after several years, the "end stage" with the so-called true "honeycombing" [24]. Both thin and thick walled cysts are mixed with normal lung tissue, fibrosis, areas of loss of lung volume [21] and may have the aspect of "ground-glass" opacities (fig. 15). In such circumstances, when performed at the same time, gallium-67 scintigraphy and CT-scan demonstrate the same peripheral, inferior and dorsal distribution of active inflammatory lesions. In PSS, honeycombing may occur in the central area of

the lungs (fig. 15), as the typical triangular pattern of gallium-67 uptake demonstrates on posterior chest scintigraphy (fig. 16).

As disease distribution cannot be assessed from the conventional chest X-rays, and as HRCT-scan provides optimal visualization of the lung in fibrosis alveolitis, gallium-67 scintigraphy can be used as a sensitive indicator of disease activity. Both gallium-67 scintigraphy and regional DTPA-99mTc clearance rate measurement could depict abnormalities in asymptomatic patients leading to proper monitoring of early therapy [25, 26]

Lymphocytic interstitial pneumonitis (LIP), first

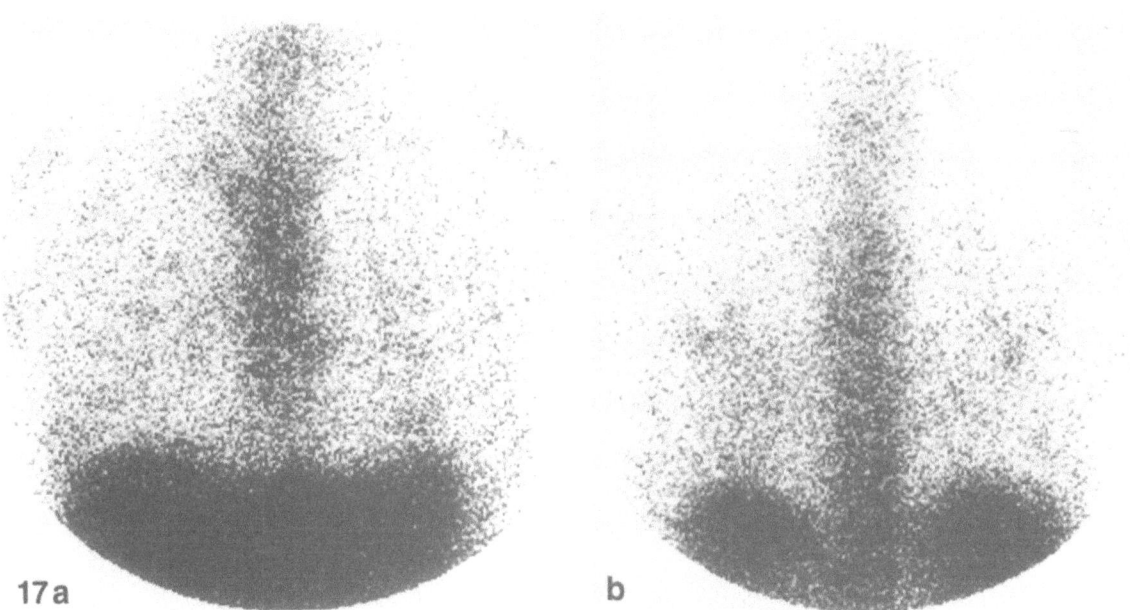

Fig. 17 a, b. Gallium-67 scintigraphy in lymphocytic interstitial pneumonitis (LIP): non-significant tracer uptake, weak and diffuse in the lung bases with intense activity in the bone marrow, liver and spleen related to the systemic involvement of the inflammatory disease. **a** Anterior and **b** posterior views of the chest

described in 1966 by Liebow and Carrington, is characterized by diffuse infiltration of the lung interstitium by small, noncleaved lymphocytes and plasma cells.

Chest X-ray demonstrates reticulonodular infiltrates of the bases similar to those seen in UIP, and also poorly circumscribed alveolar, micronodular, "downy" opacities. Therefore, in the absence of fibrosis and in spite of clinical evidence, such as chest radiograph and often even CT-scan, gallium-67 scintigraphy is almost negative or demonstrates a mild, diffuse, peripheral enhancement. This situation is nearly always found in SLE (fig. 17). A high, diffuse, homogeneous uptake of gallium-67 in the whole lung would more probably suggest infectious disease or lymphoma.

Alveolar Hemorrhage (AH) is a rare complication of connective tissue disease and pulmonary vasculitis. It is usually severe, often undetected and acutely progressive [27].Chest X-rays reveal a fluffy alveolar infiltrate which is usually bilateral. If hemorrhage recurs, fibrosis may develop, resulting in alveolar-interstitial pneumonia [27-29]. On CT, ground-glass opacities demonstrate an advanced stage of the disease. Earlier, if gallium-67 scintigraphy is performed, hemosiderin laden alveolar macrophages lead to a mild but well delineated regional uptake.

Bronchiolitis obliterans (BO) is defined by histologic features and may be pure [30, 31], with no parenchymal lesions, or associated with intraalveolar fibrosis which is difficult to differentiate from UIP, or organizing pneumonia [32].

Certain types of bronchiolitis are observed following exposure to toxic fumes, administration of D-penicillamine or after organ transplantation [33]. Chest X-ray and CT-scan in pure forms of BO contribute little. The diagnosis is difficult to assess and can hardly be made in the absence of histologic findings in the small bronchi or bronchioles. Gallium-67 scintigraphy is negative.

These four pulmonary and/or bronchial complications may occur in the course of SLE, nevertheless AH and pure BO are most frequent.

UIP is the most common pulmonary complication in PSS. It may reveal the disease. It occurs most often in the course of recognized PSS and may be diagnosed early by CT-scan, bronchoalveolar lavage and scintigraphy. UIP predisposes to bronchial or bronchoalveolar carcinoma.

Besides the classic pleural effusion, which contains little glucose, the main complications of RA are interstitial pneumonitis, necrobiotic nodules, Caplan's syndrome, and BO. RA is one of the connective tissue diseases which carries the highest risk of pure bronchiolitis obliterans, but most patients with RA who develop this complication are treated with D-penicillamine.

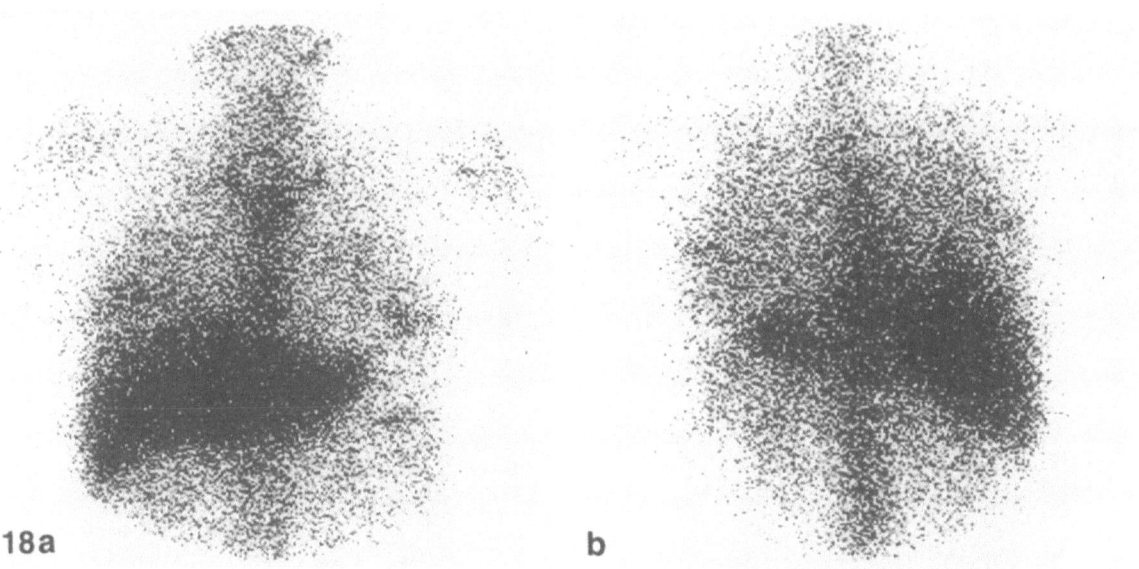

Fig. 18 a, b. Diffuse uptake of gallium-67 in the posterobasal area of the lung with some heterogeneous foci of activity in interstitial pneumonitis occurring in the course of Sjögren syndrome. In SS this pattern seems to be related to a heterogeneous distribution of the systemic lesions. **a** Anterior and **b** posterior views of the chest

In Sjögren's syndrome (SS), possible association of interstitial pneumonitis with a restrictive syndrome was initially described [34] (fig. 18). It involves 10% of patients. The occurrence of B lymphoma is especially serious in the presence of LIP. Possible involvement of large bronchi was then studied, which causes an obstructive syndrome, above all bronchiolitis obliterans [35].

Polymyositis-Dermatomyositis (PDM) is essentially an UIP, which in certain prospective series represented more than 50% of cases, but which cause troublesome clinical manifestations in less than 10% of cases. Bronchoalveolar lavage and gallium-67 scintigraphy can assist in the follow-up of these patients and in adjustment of therapy [36]. When SS and PDM are associated at the end stage disease, they can lead to a complex, severe cardiopulmonary impairment which might need graft surgery. At this stage, gallium-67 scintigraphy is almost negative because the fibrosis is established and no longer expresses activity. Nevertheless, the CT-scan shows extensive, extremely dense fibrosis, bronchiectasis, cystic destructive impairment and subpleural lines. This is evocative of centrolobular fibrosis.

Diffuse interstitial lung diseases with known etiologies

Pneumoconioses

Pneumoconioses are produced by the inhalation of inorganic dust. These dusts may be fibrous minerals (asbestos, talc), nonfibrous mineral (silica, coal) or metal (beryllium). In addition to pulmonary fibrosis and benign pleural disease there is a five fold increase in the rate of bronchogenic carcinoma among nonsmoking asbestos workers when compared to a nonsmoking control population. Deposition of coal dust around respiratory bronchioles causes symptoms or measurable physiological problems in most workers. In silicosis, the course of the disease may be modified by other factors such as superinfection and careful and repeated search for mycobacterial disease is mandatory, especially with sudden worsening of the condition.

Simple pneumoconiosis consists of a fine diffuse reticulonodular pattern seen on chest roentgenogram. This can eventually result in progressive massive fibrosis and restrictive lung disease.The chest X-ray findings do not correlate well with the symptomatology and physiological impairment. More extensive significant, intense accumulation of gallium-67 occurs (fig. 19) than could have been estimated from radiographic abnormalities [37]. Gallium-67 scanning may be useful in studies of the activity and progression of the disease as no specific treatment exists for any pneumoconiosis.

The pathogenesis of berylliosis is very different from that of the other fibrogenic pneumoconioses. Reaction to beryllium is systemic and involves an immune response with granuloma formation. In acute

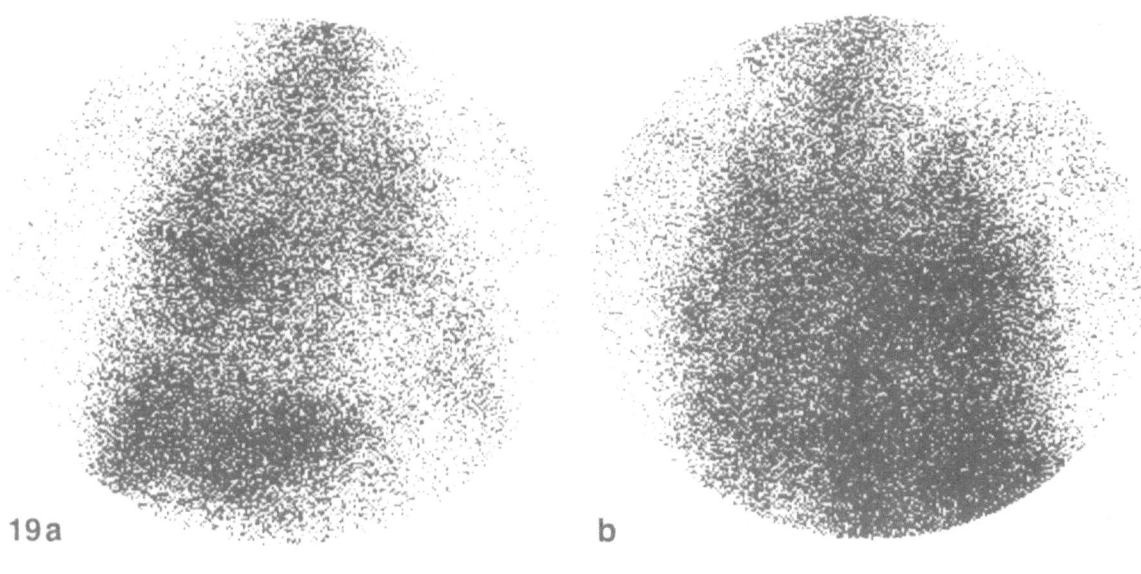

19a   b

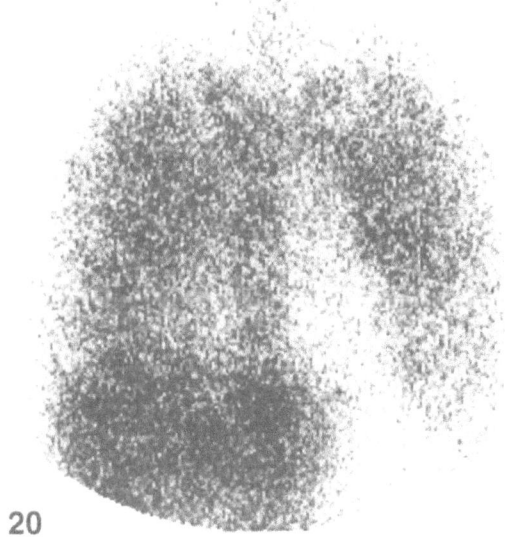

20

Fig. 19 a, b. Coal worker's pneumoconiosis: uptake of gallium-67 in the whole lung with a large intense accumulation in the center of the right lung leading to the suspicion of complicated pneumoconiosis. **a** Anterior and **b** posterior views of the chest

Fig. 20. Acute berylliosis in a patient working in the aerospace industry. The diffuse gallium-67 uptake involve the whole lung (anterior view). The relatively high bone marrow uptake is related to the systemic reaction to beryllium

berylliosis, diffuse bilateral consolidation may be seen on chest X-ray. This reflects diffuse alveolar damage also associated with a severe, biexponential increase in the DTPA clearance rate similar to that of adult respiratory distress syndrome (ARDS) and a diffuse significant thoracic uptake of gallium-67 (fig. 20). Chronic berylliosis simulates sarcoidosis and sometimes the other pneumoconioses such as asbestosis. When extensive interstitial fibrosis is present, the appearance is indistinguishable from other known causes of parenchymal fibrosis.

Hypersensitivity pneumonitis

Hypersensitivity pneumonitis or extrinsic allergic alveolitis occurs in individuals who have developed an abnormal sensitivity to some organic agent. The most prevalent antigens are thermophilic actinomycetes

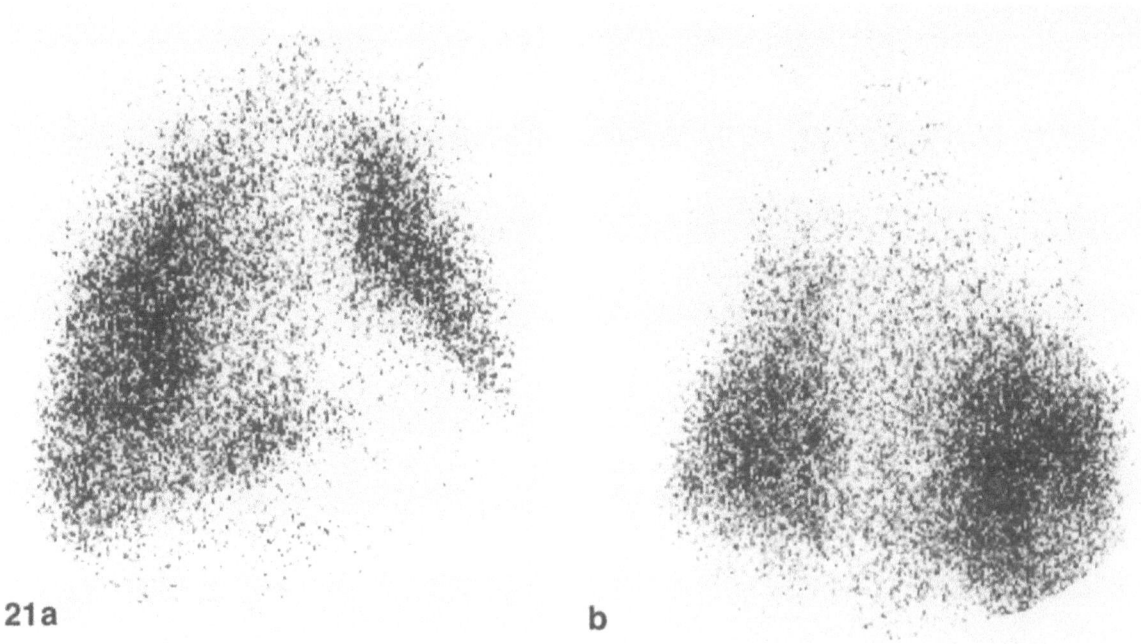

Fig. 21 a, b. Bird-breeder's lung at the acute phase of allergic alveolitis: The uptake of gallium-67 is intense and diffuse but the usual sparing of the apices is clearly shown on the two views. **a** Anterior and **b** posterior views

(farmer's lung) and avium serum proteins (bird-breeder's lung).

About six hours following exposure, X-ray can reveal nodular or reticulonodular infiltrates with relative sparing of the apices. However the chest radiograph may be normal in spite of significant symptoms. Bronchoalveolar lavage yields abnormally large numbers of T-lymphocytes, particularly T-suppressor cells. The duration of symptoms may gradually increase with repeated exposure and eventually results in the development of pulmonary fibrosis and restrictive lung disease.

In spite of the findings of a normal radiograph, gallium-67 scintigraphy demonstrates intense diffuse lung uptake related to the early detection of interstitial inflammatory reaction (fig. 21). With the development of interstitial fibrosis, radiographic and scintigraphic patterns may be indistinguishable from the many other causes of interstitial fibrosis.

Macrophage scintigraphy

In view of their early involvement in inflammatory diseases, macrophages are a privileged target for a functional approach to lesions by scintigraphic imaging. The concept of such macrophage targeting

was initially developed both to attempt to detect whether there was an active inflammatory component which could be treated and also to assess subsequently the patient's response to such therapy. In addition, a functional approach to inflammation at the cellular level was considered in order to provide a tool for the evaluation of the activity and evolutivity of the pathology. However, such a functional approach requires careful assessment both from the point of view of the strategy itself and of the instrinsic performance of the targeting agent used.

J001X is a natural acylated poly-galactoside of bacterial origin isolated from membranes of a non-encapsulated and non-pathogenic strain of Klebsiella pneumoniae. This fully characterized agent of 34 kDa molecular weight has been demonstrated to bind macrophage-monocyte cell lineages selectively and in vitro studies have shown that CD11b/CD18 and CD14 are involved in this interaction [38].

Optimization of J001X has been achieved to reduce the immunopharmacological activity mainly for macrophage activation and cytokine secretion to an almost negligible level, while preserving its targeting properties [39]. Due to its molecular structure and amphiphatic properties, this technetium-99m labeled

Fig. 22 a-c. Sarcoidosis: lymph node involvement. **a** A posteroanterior roentgenogram of this 48-year-old asymptomatic man, reveals marked enlargement of both hila. The lungs are clear; **b** anterior J001X scintigraphy 3h after inhalation reveals the mediastinal uptake corresponding exactly to the gallium mediastinal pattern; **c** anterior thoracic gallium scan 48h after injection: note bilateral mediastinal fixation and the gallium uptake in the liver

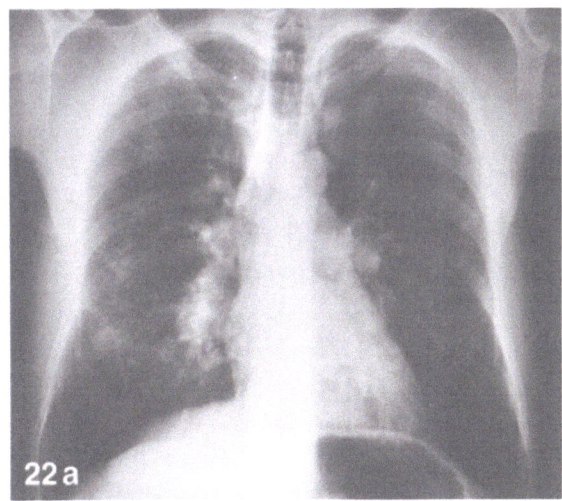

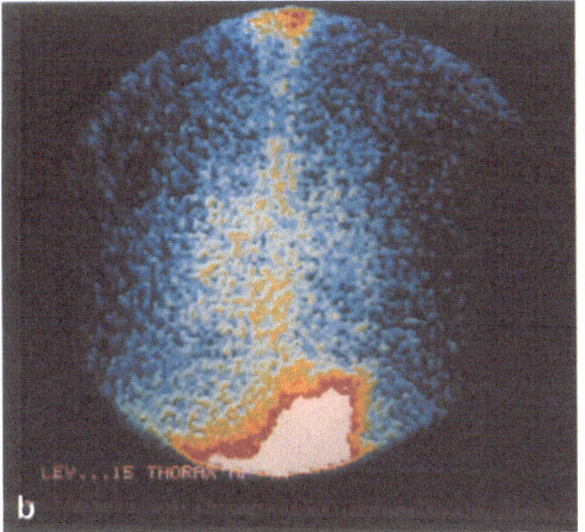

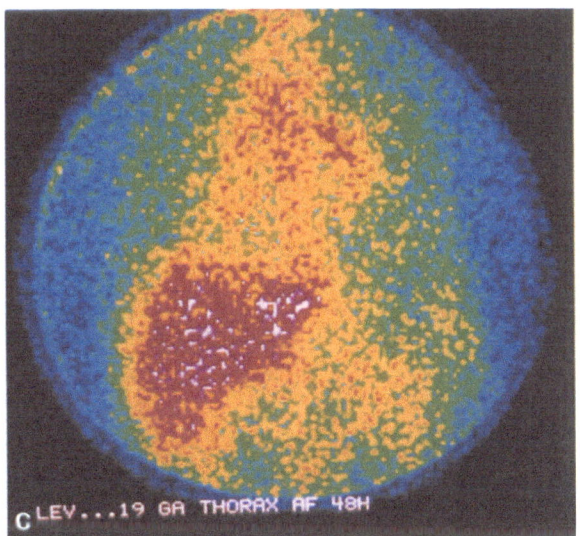

agent with exhibits high diffusibility in tissues resulting in efficient targeting of lesions recruiting macrophages that have been visualized with high contrast in a variety of experimental models [40, 41].When inhaled as an aerosol of large size particles (5-13 nm) using an ultrasound TV 6000 (Siemens) nebulizer, technetium-99m-J001X is absorbed through the respiratory tract and rapidly diffuses in blood, lymph and extracellular spaces.

Practically, 1 mg J001X is labeled with 1 110 MBq of technetium-99m then patients inhale the aerosol for 15 minutes in an especially devised aspiration hood. They wear gloves and protective clothing that are changed after inhalation and before each scintigraphic acquisition to avoid skin contamination which could result in false positive foci.

Anterior and posterior images are recorded on a 128 x 128 matrix both 3 and 5 hours after inhalation [42]. For interpretation, digitized contrast enhancement is performed by scaling the maximum of intensity to a lower value than the maximum count. The scintigraphy is considered as normal when no activity is detectable in the lung, hilar regions or mediastinum on acquisitions performed 5 hours after inhalation. For abnormal fixing foci, an uptake index is systematically determined referring the mean count in these areas to the non-specific activity counted in a reference area over the shoulder.

In the first study, J001X scintigraphy was performed in 22 patients with sarcoidosis and compared with gallium-67 scanning in 10 of them. Seven patients representing 3 stages of disease were positive in both tests (figs. 22, 23).

From a subsequent multicenter trial of 91 patients with sarcoidosis, bilateral pulmonary fixation was observed in 38 (42%). Lung fixation was observed in

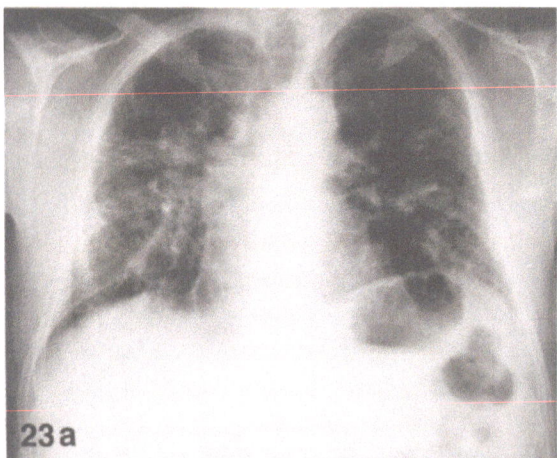

Fig. 23. Sarcoidosis: pulmonary involvement. **a** Postero-anterior roentgenogram of this 37-year-old man reveals patchy opacities in both lungs, predominantly situated in central lung regions. This man complained of exertional dyspnea; **b** posterior J001X scintigraphy 3h after inhalation: diffuse pulmonary fixation; **c** posterior gallium scan 48h after injection: note diffuse pulmonary fixation and physiologic gallium uptake in the liver

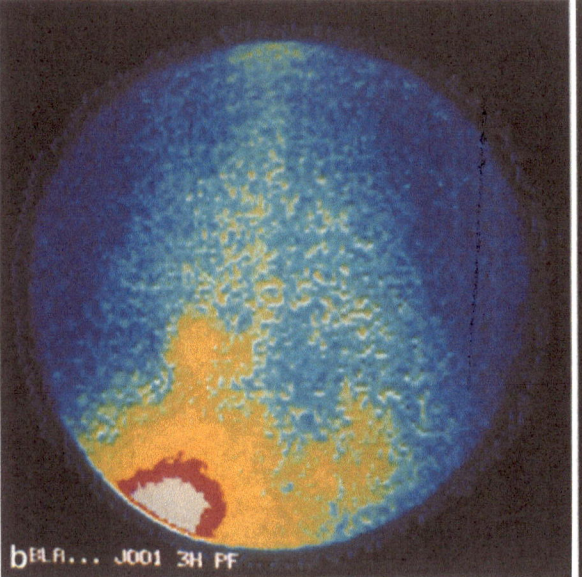

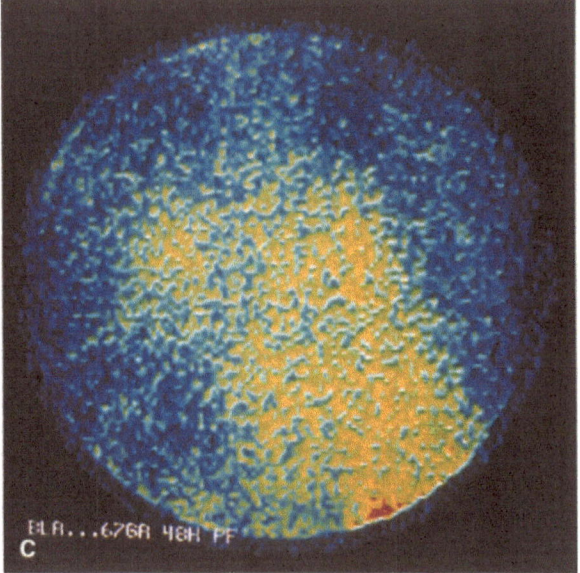

stage 0 or 1 patients apparently without parenchymal involvement, whereas few pulmonary fixations were observed in stage 2 or 3 patients. Comparison with gallium-67 scans in the same patients supports evidence that information provided by these two scintigraphic methods is different, this observation being reinforced when the comparison was focused on markers of severity of the disease. Indeed, patients with functional impairment (decreased DLCO) had lung J001X uptake in less than 40% of cases, and fixed gallium in almost 80%; patients with normal PFT were more frequently J001X positive than those with functional impairment.

In other words, patients with positive J001X and negative gallium scintigraphy mostly have a non-fibrosing interstitial syndrome and BAL lymphocytes, without functional impairment and increased SACE.

In occupational lung diseases, 28 patients with professional dust exposure were explored by J001X. The interstitial lesions were a restrictive syndrome in 6 cases of 28, decreased DLCO in 9 of 25 and a radiological interstitial syndrome in 11 of 26.

Patients with fully developed disease and severe functional impairment had negative J001X scintigraphy corresponding to extinction of the inflammatory process. The interstitial impairment was associated with positive J001X scintigraphy. Patients without known interstitial lesions mostly had negative J001X scintigraphy confirming the absence of parenchymal disorders. In some patients, pulmonary uptake of J001X revealing an early inflammatory process could predict future respiratory deterioration.

The scintigraphic behavior of J001X in cryptogenic fibrosing alveolitis was documented in 12 patients. All the patients with lung uptake (42% of cases) presented a frosted glass aspect on CT scan while patients with negative J001X scintigraphy had fibrosis on HRCT, with restrictive syndrome and diffusion capacity impairment.

Lung exploration with J001X scintigraphy in systemic diseases was performed in 54 patients with scleroderma, rheumatoid arthritis and lupus and led to bilateral lung uptake in 31% of cases. All patients with fibrosis on HRCT had negative J001X scintigraphy and lung uptake was noted when interstitial syndrome without signs of fibrosis was present.

In conclusion, data from 156 patients with interstitial lung disease indicate that J001X scintigraphy provides information that is complementary to gallium scintigraphy and radiological examination. At equal stages of evaluation, positive J001X scintigraphy should indicate the presence or persistence of an active inflammatory process. Therefore, whether positive or negative, J001X scintigraphy appears to be informative:

– positive in the presence of active lung disease or in the case of persistence of active foci;

– negative, if no parenchymal lesions are present, in the case of cured disease or resulting from the extinction of the process such as in fibrosis.

These potentials of J001X scintigraphy remain to be confirmed in a larger series of patients including follow-up studies for the assessment of the predictive value of this new scintigraphic strategy.

^{99m}Tc-DTPA scintigraphy

All physiological or pathological processses, such as enlargement of the intercellular pores of the pulmonary epithelium, surfactant change, modification of alveolar surface tension, etc. which can modify the factors influencing the transmembrane passage of ^{99m}Tc-DTPA, can alter the half-life of the radiotracer.

Increase in the pulmonary clearance of ^{99m}Tc-DTPA is observed after even very small changes of the alveolocapillary membrane. Non-smokers exposed to tobacco intoxication show a higher pulmonary clearance of ^{99m}Tc-DTPA. This acceleration is related more to the intensity of the intoxication than to its duration. The clearance of ^{99m}Tc-DTPA returns to normal values 3-4 weeks after the intoxication.

The first studies were carried out in patients with idiopathic interstitial pulmonary fibrosis and it was found that the pulmonary clearance of DTPA was accelerated in this disease. Later numerous studies evaluating the pulmonary clearance of ^{99m}Tc-DTPA

were carried out in various pathological conditions such as collagen diseases (Goodpasture syndrome, lupus erythematosus, rheumatoid arthritis, scleroderma, Sjögren's syndrome), sarcoidosis pneumoconiosis and radiation-caused lung disease. They demonstrated the possibilities of the diagnosis of pulmonary lesions [46]. The following conclusions can be drawn from these results:

The pulmonary clearance of ^{99m}Tc-DTPA is a method which is very sensitive in the detection of pulmonary interstitial lesions.

The diagnostic sensitivity of the method is greater than that of chest X-ray, diffusion tests and arterial blood gas measurements (fig. 24).

The test of pulmonary clearance of DTPA is, however, without etiological specificity since clearance changes in various conditions affecting the lungs.

Changes in DTPA pulmonary clearance can be observed without any respiratory symptoms and signs (clinical or radiological). These changes permit the early identification of the etiology of the lesion by more invasive methods.

Absolute values of acceleration of the pulmonary clearance of DTPA are related to the degree of cellular infiltration of the interstitium and have a prognostic importance.

Serial determination of the clearance of ^{99m}Tc-DTPA from the lungs can be used to trace the progression of pulmonary lesions or treatment efficacy.

The pulmonary clearance of ^{99m}Tc-DTPA is accelerated in acute respiratory distress syndrome. In hemodynamic pulmonary edema it remains normal for a long time. In chronic obstructive bronchopneumopathies the pulmonary clearance of DTPA is not accelerated.

The study of the pulmonary clearance of ^{99m}Tc-DTPA is particulary interesting in patients with HIV infection.

The results may be pathologic at the stage of lymphocytic alveolitis (the half-life of clearance being correlated with the absolute lymphocyte count), particularly in Pneumocystis carinii infections. Moderate acceleration of pulmonary clearance may be a sign of infection, (P. carinii, cytomegalovirus, etc), of pulmonary Kaposi sarcoma, of lymphocytic alveolitis or pulmonary lymphoma. Very high acceleration (with a half-life of 10-20 minutes) with a biexponential elimination curve is highly suggestive of P. carinii infection. Whatever the etiology, the pulmonary DTPA clearance can reveal lung

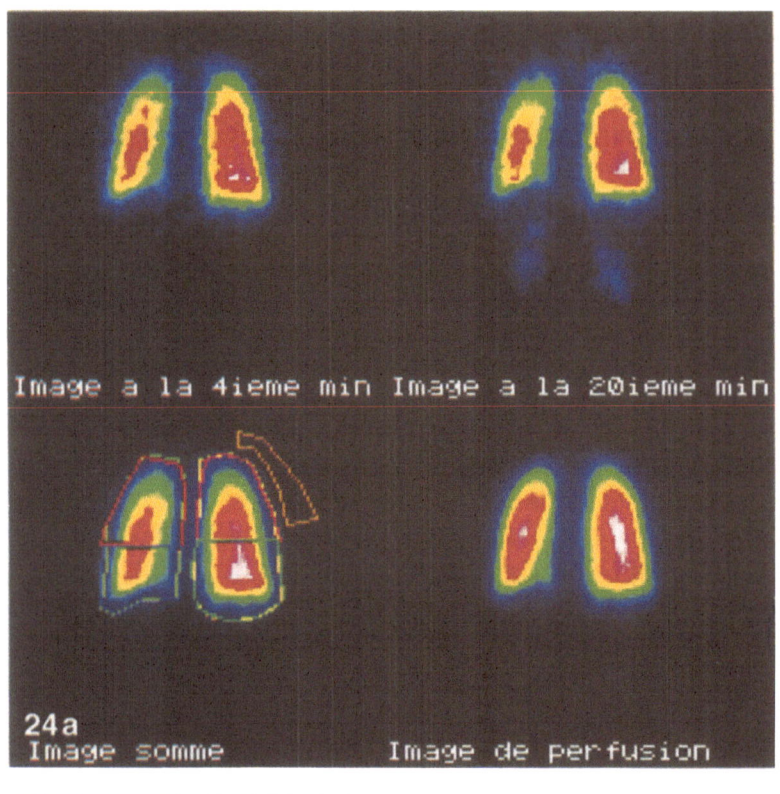

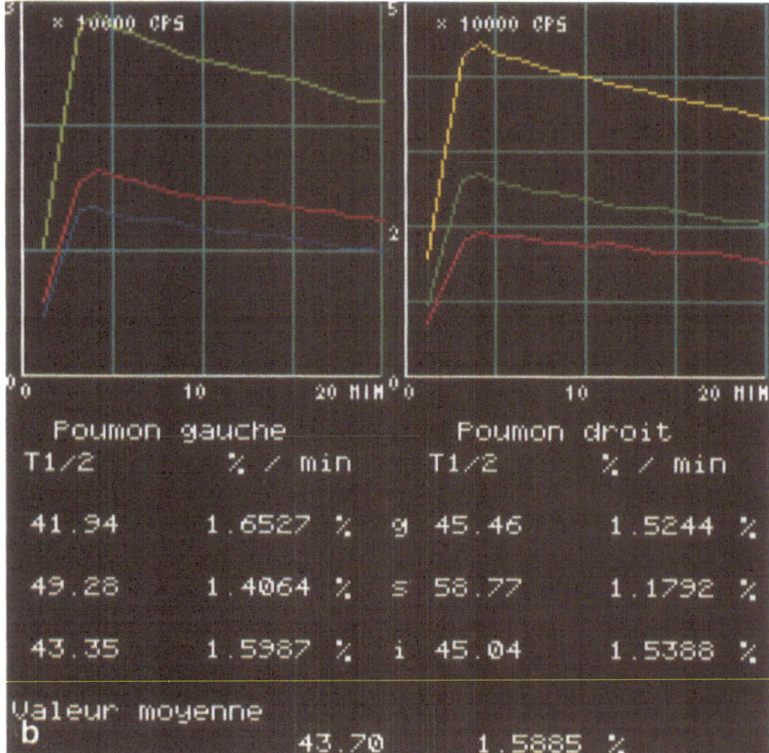

Fig. 24 a, b. In 1991 this patient was treated with steroids for eosinophilia pneumoniae. At this time 99mTc-DTPA lung clearance was abnormal (T1/2 = 28 min). Since June 1992 the patient has received no therapy. **a, b** In October 1992, chest X-ray, thoracic CT, 99mTc-DTPA lung clearance were normal. However pulmonary function tests demonstrated a restrictive syndrome. The patient remained without therapy and 8 months later a new check up showed no evidence of disease

involvement, often before other diagnostic methods can demonstrate it. It may also be an indication to perform broncho-fibroscopy to elucidate etiology.

The study of pulmonary clearance of ^{99m}Tc-DTPA during the follow-up of HIV-infected subjects can thus help in the detection of complications in the subclinical stage and in the evaluation of the efficacy of therapeutic methods used to control pulmonary involvement.

Whatever the clinical indication for which the pulmonary ^{99m}Tc-DTPA clearance test was performed, the possibility of tobacco intoxication must be always considered in the interpretation and follow-up.

The determination of the pulmonary clearance of ^{99m}Tc-DTPA, bearing in mind the technical problems and the interpretation of the results in which the possible influence of smoking must also be considered, has an unquestionable clinical value. Although clearance was a low value for the diagnosis of the etiology, it is highly sensitive in the demonstration of lung involvement.

References

1. De Remee RA (1987) Diffuse interstitial pulmonary disease from the perspective of the clinician. Chest 92 : 1068-1073
2. Cherniack RM, Crystal RG, Kalica AR (1991) Current concepts in idiopathic pulmonary fibrosis : a road map for the future. Am Rev Respir Dis 143 : 680-683
3. Tsan MF (1985) Mechanism of Gallium-67 accumulation in inflammatory lesions. J Nucl Med 26 : 88-92
4. Okhubo Y, Sawamura H, Katoh S, Sasayama A, Abe K, Kohno H, Kubodera A (1990) Studies on Gallium-67 uptake by mouse granuloma tissues. Nucl Med Biol 18 : 205-208
5. Hoffer P (1980) Gallium : Mechanisms. J Nucl Med 21 : 282-285
6. Bekerman C, Hoffer PB, Bitran JD, Gupta RG (1980) Gallium-67 citrate imaging studies of the lung. Sem Nucl Med 10 : 286-301
7. Sulavik SB, Spencer RP, Weed DA, Shapiro HR, Shiue ST, Castriotta RJ (1990) Recognition of distinctive patterns of Gallium-67 distribution in sarcoidosis. J Nucl Med 31 : 1909-1914
8. Gupta RG, Bekerman C, Sicilian L, Oparil S, Pinsky SM, Szidon JP (1982) Gallium-67 citrate scanning and serum angiotensin converting enzyme levels in sarcoidosis. Radiology 144 : 895-899
9. Klech H, Köhn H, Kummer F, Mostbeck A (1982) Assessment of activity in sarcoidosis. Chest 82 : 732-738
10. Köhn H, Klech H, Mostbeck A, Kummer F (1982) Gallium-67 scanning for assessment of disease activity and therapy decisions in pulmonary sarcoidosis in com-parison to chest scintigraphy, serum ACE and blood T-lymphocytes. Eur J Nucl Med 7 : 413-416
11. Nosal A, Schleissner LA, Mishkin FS (1979) Angio-tensin-I-converting enzyme and Gallium scan in non-invasive evaluation of sarcoidosis. Ann Intern Med 90 : 328-331
12. Gupta RG, Bekerman C, Catchatourian R et al (1979) Relationship between bronchoalveolar cellular analysis and Gallium-67 citrate uptake in active sarcoidosis (abstr). Clin Res 27 : 622A
13. Baughman RP, Fernandez M, Bosken CH, Mantil J, Hurtubise P (1984) Comparison of Gallium-67 scanning, bronchoalveolar lavage and serum angiotensin-conver-ting enzyme levels in pulmonary sarcoidosis. Am Rev Respir Dis 129 : 676-681
14. Klech H, Köhn H, Huppmann M, Pohl W (1987) Thoracic imaging with Gallium-67. Eur J Nucl Med 13 : S24-S36
15. Van Unnik JG, van Royen EA, Alberts C, van der Schott JB (1983) A method of quantitative Gallium-67 scinti-graphy in the evaluation of pulmonary sarcoidosis. Eur J Nucl Med 8 : 351-353
16. Bourguet P, Delaval Ph, Herry JY (1986) Direct quanti-tation of thoracic Gallium-67 uptake in sarcoidosis. J Nucl Med 27 : 1550-1556
17. Crystal RG, Bitterman PB, Rennard DI, Hance AJ, Keogh BA (1984). Interstitial lung diseases of unknown cause. Disorders characterized by chronic inflammation of the lower respiratory tract. N Engl J Med 310 : 154-166, 235-244
18. Epler GR, McLoud TC, Gaensler EA, Mikus JP, Carrington CB (1978). Normal chest roentgenograms in chronic diffuse infiltration lung disease. N Engl J Med 298 : 934-939
19. Watters LC, Schwartz MI, Cherniack RM (1987) Idio-pathic pulmonary fibrosis. Pretreatment bronchoalveolar lavage cellular constituants and their relationships with histopathology and clinical response to therapy. Am Rev Respir 135 : 696-704
20. Stoller JK, Rankin JA, Reynolds HY (1987) The impact of broncho-alveolar lavage cell analysis on clinician's diagnostic reasoning about interstitial lung diseases. Chest 92 : 839-843
21. Muller NL, Staples CA, Miller RR, Vedal S, Thurlbeck WM, Ostrow DN (1987) Disease activity in idiopathic pulmonary fibrosis : computed tomography-pathologic correlation. Radiology 165 : 731-734
22. Grenier P, Valeyre D, Cluzel P, Brauner MW, Lenoir S, Chastang C (1991) Chronic diffuse infiltration lung disease : assessment of diagnostic value of chest radio-graphy and high-resolution CT. Radiology 179 : 123-132
23. Begin CJ, Müller NL (1985) CT in the diagnosis of inter-stitial lung disease. A J R 145 : 505-510
24. Genereux GP (1975) The end stage lung. Pathogenesis, pathology, and radiology. Radiology 116 : 279-289
25. Caillat-Vigneron N, Moretti JL, Valeyre D, Le Guludec D, Sadoun D, Battesti JP (1990) Pulmonary epithelial

permeability versus 67Ga uptake in chronic interstitial lung disease (CILD) (abstr). Eur J Nucl Med 16 : S150

26. Harrison NK, Glanville AR, Strickland B, Haslam PL, Corrin B, Addis BJ, Lawrence R, Millar AB, Black CM, Turner-Warwick M (1987) Pulmonary involvement in systemic sclerosis : the detection of early changes by thin section CT scan, bronchoalveolar lavage and ^{99m}Tc-DTPA clearence. Respir Med 83 : 403-414

27. Leatherman JW, Davies SF, Hoidal JR (1984) Alveolar hemorrhage syndromes : diffuse microvascular lung hemorrhage in immune and idiopathic disorders. Medicine 63 : 343-361

28. Bonnotte B, Chantereau MJ, Lorcerie B, Chauffert B, Noblet JF, Chalopin JM, Martin F (1992) Hemmorragies intra-alvéolaires au cours des maladies systémiques. Presse Med 21 : 839-842

29. Leatherman JW (1987) Immune alveolar haemorrhage. Chest 91 : 891-897

30. Macklem PT, Thurlbeck WM, Fraser RG (1971) Chronic obstructive disease in small airways. Ann Intern Med 74 : 167-177

31. Epler GR, Colby TV (1983) The spectrum of bronchiolitis obliterans. Chest 83 : 161-162

32. Cordier JF, Loire R, Peyrol S (1991) Bronchiolitis obliterans organizing pneumonia. Originalité et limites d'une entité anatomo-clinique. Rev Mal Resp 8 : 139-152

33. Cordier JF, Moulin J, Brune J, Moulin G, Touraine R (1981) Accidents respiratoires au cours de traitements par la D Pénicillamine : alévolites et bronchiolites. Rev Fr Mal Resp 9 : 319-326

34. Strimlan CV, Rosenow EC, Divertie MB (1976) Pulmonary manifestations of Sjögren's syndrome. Chest 70 : 354-361

35. Newball HD, Brahim SA (1977) Chronic obstructive airway disease in patients with Sjögren's syndrome. Am Rev Resp Dis 115 : 295-304

36. Schwartz MI, Matthay RA, Sahn SA, Stanford RE, Mamorstein BL, Scheinlorn DF (1976) Interstitial disease in polymyositis and dermatomyositis : an analysis of 6 cases and review of the literature. Medicine 55 : 89-104

37. Siemsen JK, Sargent EN, Grebe SF, Winsor DW, Wentz D, Jacobsen G (1974) Pulmonary concentration of Gallium-67 in pneumoconiosis. Am J Roentgenol Radium Ther Nuc Med 120 : 815-820

38. Hmama Z, Normier G, Kouassi E, Flacher M, Binz H, Revillard JP, (1992) Binding of a membrane proteoglycan from Klebsiella pneumoniae and its chemically-defined derivatives to human leukocytes. Immunobiology (in press)

39. Hmama Z, Lina G, Normier G, Binz H, Revillard JP (1992) Monocyte cytokine secretion induced by chemically-defined derivatives of Klebsiella pneumoniae. Clin Exp Immunol (in press)

40. Perrin F, Pittet JC, Hoffschir D, Normier G, Binz H, Le Pape A, (1993) Scintigraphic potential of J001X acylated poly-galactoside for the imaging of inflammatory lesions in pigs. Nucl Med Biol (in press)

41. Diot P, Le Pape A, Nolibe D, Normier G, Binz H, Revillard JP, Lasfargues G, Lavandier M, Lemarié E (1992) Scintigraphy with J001X, a Klebsiella membrane glycolipopeptide, for the early diagnosis of chronic berylliosis. Results in an experimental model of berylliosis in baboons. Br J Ind Med 49 : 359-364

42. Diot P, Lemarie E, Baulieu JL, Pascal S, Vaillant L, Revillard JP, Binz H, Normier G, Le Pape A, (1992) Scintigraphy with J001X macrophage targeting glycolipopeptide : a new approach for sarcoidosis imaging. Chest 102 : 670-676

43. Chinet T, Dusser D, Labrune S, Collignon MA, Chretien J, Huchon G (1981) Lung function declines in patients with pulmonary sarcoidosis and increased respiratory epithelial permeability to ^{99m}Tc-DTPA. Am Rev Respir Dis 141 : 445-449

44. Mason GR, Uszler JM, Effros RM, Reid E (1983) Rapidly reversible alterations of pulmonary epithelial permeability induced by smoking. Chest 1 : 6-11

45. Oberdorster G, Utell MJ, Morrow PE, Hyde RW, Weber DA (1986). Bronchial and alveolar absorption of inhaled ^{99m}Tc-DTPA. Am Rev Respir Dis 134 : 944-950

46. Rinderknecht J, Shapiro L, Krauthammer M et al (1980) Accelerated clearance of small solutes from the lungs in interstitial lung disease. Am Rev Respir Dis 121 : 105-117

Lung tumors

JL Baulieu, P Bourguet, B Desrues and E Lemarié

Introduction

In 1992 lung cancer was the most common cause of cancer death in men in the Western world, and its incidence among women is rapidly increasing. Early diagnosis and surgical intervention offers the best opportunity for survival. Unfortunately, approximately 75-80% of all lung cancers are unresectable at initial diagnosis, and more than 50% of these have metastases beyond the mediastinal nodes. Therapeutic results have been stagnant, with only a minimal increase in five-year survival during the past two decades. About 20% of the patients live for 1 year, and less than 15% survive for 5 years. The majority of lung cancers fall into four histologic types: small cell and squamous cell lung cancer, adenocarcinoma and large cell carcinoma.

The treatment of patients with small cell lung cancer is quite different from that of patients with squamous cell cancer, large cell cancer or adeno-carcinoma of the lung, cancers collectively termed non-small cell carcinomas. Small cell lung cancer accounts for 20% of the primary lung carcinomas. It can rarely be cured by surgical resection, because two-thirds of patients have clinically detectable distant metastases at the time of diagnosis. Chemotherapy improves survival in small cell lung cancer. Association of radiotherapy and chemotherapy can even cure a small fraction of patients with limited disease.

In contrast, surgery is the treatment of choice in 25 to 30% of patients with non-small cell tumor confined to the lung (stage I or II). Another 25 to 30% of patients have locally advanced cancers that extend to mediastinal or supraclavicular lymph nodes or mediastinal organs and pleura (stage IIIa or IIIb). They are usually treated with radiotherapy or occasionally chemotherapy followed by surgery. Unfortunately, in 75% of patients with stage I to IIIb disease, tumor recurs in distant sites. For the remaining 40 to 50% who have stage IV non-small cell cancer at the time of diagnosis, chemotherapy with palliative symptomatic treatment is standard care. In patients with stage IV non-small cell lung cancer, the average survival is 5-8 months from the time of diagnosis.

Since no therapy is really satisfactory, more reliable and sensitive methods are necessary for the diagnostic evaluation. Three aims can be defined: detecting lung cancer, determining the operability of the patient (staging), and evaluating the response of the patient to therapy. An important point is the evaluation of mediastinal involvement since 50% of patients with non-small cell lung carcinoma have tumor spread to the mediastinum at the time of clinical detection. Conventional radiography, computed tomography and magnetic resonance imaging are non-invasive techniques that have an important role for evaluation of the mediastinal region. Unfortunately, there is no imaging modality that has sufficient sensitivity or specificity to stage the mediastinum definitively. Nevertheless, in the last decade the role of computed tomography in the evaluation of lung tumors has increased significantly. This is due to advances in image quality. The ability of conventional imaging techniques to detect tumors is usually limited for lesions less than 1 cm in diameter.

Therefore, imaging procedures such as X-ray, ultrasound, computed tomography and magnetic resonance express differences in density. Diagnostic information obtained by nuclear medicine is based on differences in concentration of radiolabeled tracers. This concentration depends on the characteristics of the tracer and the pathophysiological conditions. Therefore, nuclear imaging expresses functional characteristics of the tumor and its environment and could be complementary to anatomic imaging.

Nuclear medicine procedures for tumor localization

For 10 years, many studies have confirmed the ability of monoclonal radiolabeled antibodies (MAbs) for both diagnostic and therapeutic purposes. Another approach could be the targeting of a cell population associated with the tumor. Macrophage scintigraphy constitutes an example of this non-specific approach.

Immunoscintigraphy

Radiolabeled monoclonal antibodies (MAbs) directed against tumor antigens are potentially of great interest in cancer diagnosis. Such MAbs have already been raised against a variety of human-associated antigens and have been used for scintigraphic detection of cancers, e.g. colorectal carcinoma, pancreatic carcinoma, melanoma, ovarian carcinoma. Several MAbs have been raised against lung cancer associated antigens, but few have been used for scintigraphic detection [1]. Immunoscintigraphic techniques involve two parameters: characteristics of monoclonal antibodies and their radiolabeling and quality of expression of the antigen by neoplastic cells.

Monoclonal antibodies and their labeling

The development of the hybridoma method by Köhler and Milstein [2] was an important event that promoted production of MAbs. MAbs are able to bind oncogen products (myc, ras), tumor markers such as carcinoembryonic antigen (CEA), alphafetoprotein, ß‑HCG, neuron specific enolase, growth factors such as epidermal growth factor (EGF), bombesin, insulin-like growth factor and cellular products [3, 4].

The purity of the antibody and its molecular form can influence avidity binding. To prevent the development of human antimouse antibodies, it is possible to use chimeric antibodies in which the Fc and the common portion of the antibody are of human origin, while the variable portion is of murine origin. It is also possible to use antibody fragments such as Fab or F(ab')2 in which the Fc portion has been removed [2, 4]. These Fab and F(ab')2 fragments also have the advantage of increasing diffusion from blood to tumor due to their small size. This method is particularly useful in attempting to visualize small lesions. Moreover, removal of the Fc portion decreases the non-specific fixation due to Fc receptors in many tissues.

Optimal imaging depends on the physical half of the isotope and the characteristics of the MAbs used. Criteria have been established for suitable MAbs labeling with radionuclides for imaging and therapy [5]: availability of the radionuclide, labeling chemistry that allows stable linkage of the antibody, a clinically convenient procedure, favorable clearance properties, and low cost of the radionuclide. Quality control of MAbs products presents special challenges because they are large complex molecules produced by living cells, and possibly contaminated by residual impurities from the host cells or culture medium. In vivo stability of the radiolabeled binding to MAbs is also an important parameter to be considered.

Tumor associated antigens

Obstacles to targeting include antigenic expression and heterogeneity in biological structure at the level of different tumors. Antigens targeted by MAbs are called tumor associated antigens and not antigens specific to the tumor. Independently of their cell surface or intracytoplasmic localization, they are found in tumor cells as well as in some normal tissues. It is necessary to target antigens that are more abundant on tumor cells than on normal cells. Radiolabeled anticarcinoembryonic antigen (CEA) MAbs has been reported to allow estimation of the local tumor extension of colorectal cancer and adenocarcinoma of the lung [3, 6, 7] but it also links non-specific crossreacting antigens (NCA) which have common epitopes with CEA.

Variations in histology and antigenic structure have been demonstrated during growth in different neoplastic lesions [8]. Diagnostic imaging of metastases can be difficult because of the lack of antigen expression in these metastatic lesions. Significant changes in radiocompound at different times have been demonstrated: MAbs are more reactive during the S phase of the cell cycle [9, 10].

Factors that affect biodistribution must be considered. These include route of administration, amount of dose, associated metobolic disorders, poor vascularity of the tumor and necrosis. In summary, a relationship exists between radioantibody uptake and tumor parameters such as the amount of the antigen expressed, tumor size, oxygen levels, presence of biological barriers and the vascular environment of the tumor [11].

Immunoscintigraphy in lung cancer

Immunoscintigraphy with radiolabeled monoclonal antibodies is a multistep procedure. Within 48 hours after IV injection one can observe high vascular activity, particularly in the mediastinum, which does not allow any imaging study. The length of this vascular activity depends especially on the size of the antibody. The use of a small form of antibody enables a more rapid clearance of radioactively-labeled antibody from background nontarget tissues, thus raising the localisation index, but the magnitude of uptake in the tumor is decreased. Therefore, depending on the immunoglobulin or the half life of the radionuclide (technetium-99m or indium-111), immunoscintigraphy is performed between 48 and 72 hours after injection.

In the lung, it is possible to define a positive uptake as any area of radioactivity that exceeds the pulmonary background. For mediastinal lesions such as lymph nodes, the analysis is more difficult because of the remaining vascular activity. In this situation, subtraction or single photon emission computerized tomographic images (SPECT) may improve detection.

Extrathoracic uptake depends on the radionuclide used. For instance indium-111 does not allow any analysis of the liver. Therefore we can consider that any abnormal extrathoracic uptake in relation to the biodistribution of the radiocompound can be read as a lesion.

The results in lung cancer imaging, while somewhat promising, have failed to fulfill the initial expectation of the "antibody guided targeting" concept. There are many physiological barriers (passage through the vascular system, non-specific uptake, liver metabolism, immune response etc) that antibodies face in their journey toward their tumor associated antigen.

Several clinical investigations have been performed using different monoclonal antibodies (CEA, B72.3, HMFG etc) in small cell and non-small cell lung carcinoma and most of these studies have demonstrated an overall diagnostic accuracy of 70 – 80% [1]. Tumor localisation was observed in both the primary tumors and the majority of the extrathoracic lesions (bone, brain etc) in patients with lung cancers.

The procedure is well-tolerated and few side-effects like skin rash or transient hypotension have been reported in the literature during immuno-scintigraphy. Patients develop antibodies against xenogenic immunoglobulins (HAMA, human anti-mouse antibodies) in a range of 5 to 25%. The use of Fab' and F(ab)'2 fragments of immunoglobulins lowers the immunogenicity.

The assessment of mediastinal lymph nodes is important for determining therapeutic options, particularly in non-small cell lung carcinoma. Since CT scan is quite sensitive in detecting enlarged lymph nodes but has low specificity for mediastinal lymph nodes between 1 and 2 cm in size, any noninvasive procedure that could add to the accuracy of mediastinal staging would be of considerable benefit. Unfortunately, whatever the monoclonal antibody and radiolabel used, very few studies in the literature have demonstrated any decisive value of immuno-scintigraphy for the assessment of mediastinal lymph nodes in non-small cell lung carcinoma. Below 2 cm it is difficult to detect lymph nodes in the mediastinum, particularly with iodine-131 and also with indium-111. The use of SPECT and ^{99m}Tc as radiolabels could avoid this technical difficulty. The results obtained by Friedman et al [12] with the Fab' fragment of a murine IgG2b monoclonal antibody (NR-LU-10) seem interesting, with detection of lesions in 91% of cases, and 86 to 89% of patients with N2 diseases identified (44 to 57% for CT). The negative predictive value was 92% (72 to 83% for CT) in this study.

Using ^{131}I labelled MAbs Po66 for immuno-scintigraphy of human lung squamous cell carcinoma, Bourguet et al. obtained 26 true positive and 7 false positive images, among 33 patients [13]. Extrathoracic metastases were well visualized but never at a submacroscopic stage (figs. 1, 2).

A ^{99m}Tc-anti-CEA MAbs BW 431/26 has been evaluated to see whether this tracer might improve the estimation of the local spread in patients with primary adenocarcinoma of the lung [7]. Among the 11 patients studied, immunoscintigraphy identified the primary tumor clearly in 7 of them (tumor size ranging from 3 to 8 cm) but provided no additional information about intrapulmonary tumor extension compared with chest radiography.

One of the main difficulties of this technique remains the specificity of the procedure. It has been demonstrated that in some cases tumor localisation could be achieved using a non-specific antibody [14]. Furthermore Biggi et al [15] showed that nonspecific uptake of antibody was possible in non-lung cancer patients (1/1 pneumonia, 2/2 abscess, 1/2 Hodgkin's disease, 1/1 tuberculosis and 1/1 micetoma).

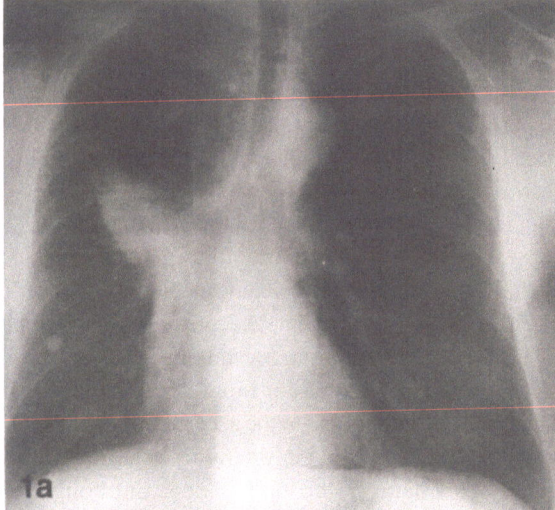
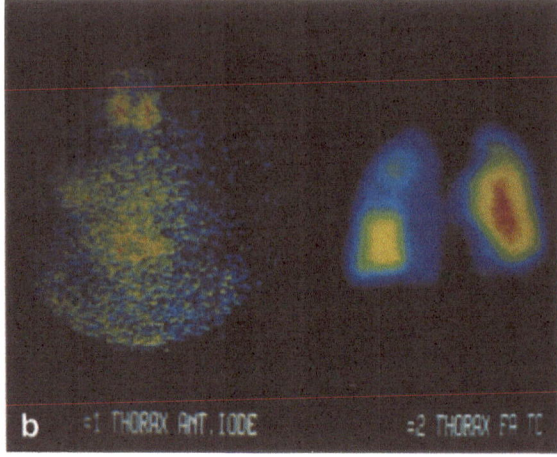

Fig. 1 a, b. Squamous cell lung carcinoma of the right upper lobe. **a** Chest X-ray, anterior view; **b** immunoscintigraphy of the same patient (left), 6 days after IV injection of iodine-131 radiolabeled monoclonal antibody Po66. Anterior view showing the tumor and also the cardiac (vascular activity) image. Scan with ^{99m}Tc radiolabeled macroaggregates (*right*) allows localization of the lungs and shows the poor vascularization of the right hilum

According to these studies, we can define the place of monoclonal antibodies in external body imaging in lung cancer. Because of the lack of specificity, this procedure is not indicated for the initial diagnosis, which is performed by complete clinical examination, chest X-rays and endoscopic investigation. On the other hand, this examination could be useful for the detection of cancer relapse or to confirm extrathoracic metastases. The lack of specificity and the difficulties of image analysis of the mediastinum do not at present allow recommendation of immunoscintigraphy as a routine procedure for accurate locoregional staging in non-small cell lung carcinoma, although the use of technetium-99m and SPECT imaging seems very encouraging [12].

A number of therapeutic trials have been undertaken using both polyclonal and monoclonal antitumor antibody radioisotope conjugates [16]. Immunoscintigraphy might determine targeted antigen tumor content before therapeutic antibody administration. Such targeted radiotherapy has been applied to patients with malignant pleural effusions [17]. This phase I study showed the disappearance of activity at a mean of 30 to 130 h while blood measurements showed that less than 10% of the radioactivity was in the circulation. In all therapeutic trials, the principal problems encountered have been the rapid development of immunity against the antibodies used

and the fact that a relatively small fraction of the total radioactivity injected is concentrated in the tumor.

Gallium scintigraphy

Due to its affinity to tumors, gallium-67 has been used in the investigation of patients with lung cancer or with primary (e.g. lymphoma) or metastatic (e.g. colorectal cancer) thoracic neoplastic disease.

Primary tumors have never been diagnosed by gallium scanning. Gallium could be taken up by nonneoplastic lesions (sarcoidosis, tuberculosis, and infectious disease) and differential diagnosis could be obtained by clinical examination, and endoscopic and radiologic investigation.

Between 1970 and 1985, tremendous amounts of data were accumulated on gallium scanning for the clinical evaluation of oncology patients (staging and recurrence evaluation). Positive gallium-67 scans are reported to occur in between 70 and 100% of patients with lung carcinoma [18]. The uptake is greater in undifferentiated carcinomas (probably due to the high associated inflammation), less in squamous cell tumors and least in adenocarcinomas. However no significant relationship between the intensity of tumor uptake and histologic cell type was found.

The false negative rate of gallium scans in patients with lung carcinoma ranges from 22 to 0%. The most

Fig. 2 a-c. Squamous cell lung carcinoma of the left upper lobe with pulmonary and cutaneous metastases. **a** Chest X-ray, anterior view. Tumor of the left upper lobe with atelectasis. The right opacity is a chest wall metastasis; **b** immunoscintigraphy with iodine-131 radiolabeled monoclonal antibody Po66 *(left)* and labeled macroaggregates *(right).* Anterior view showing the chest wall metastasis. Note that the vascular activity does not allow an accurate analysis of the mediastinum; **c** posterior view (same patient) showing the metastasis but also the tumor of the left upper lobe. The uptake in the left lower lobe is due to nodular lung metastases

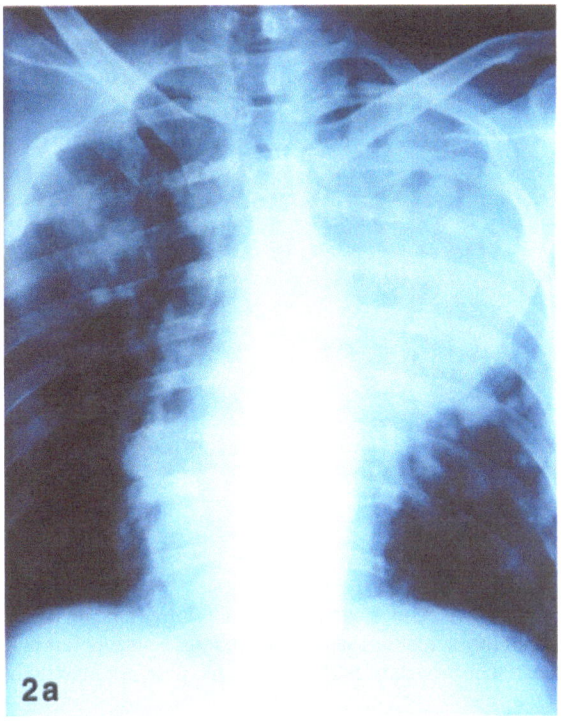

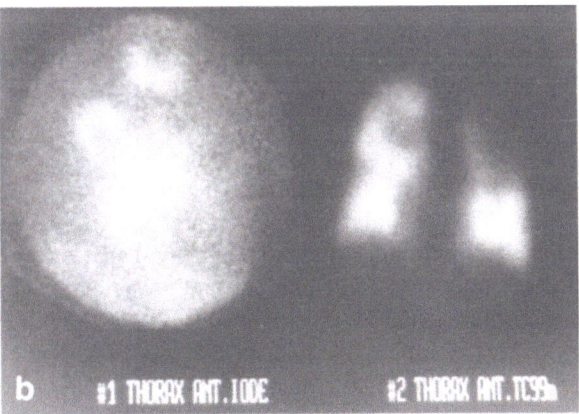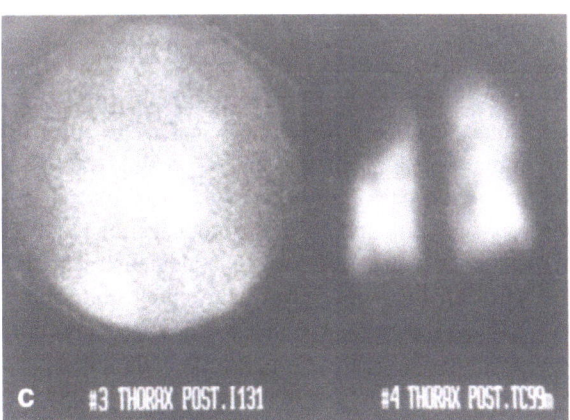

common causes of false negative findings are: tumor size less than 2 cm, hepatic activity that obscures lesions in the right lower lobe, tumor necrosis and recent administration of cytostatic drugs.

Evaluation of the mediastinum and hilar involvement is essential for prediction of operability. A value of 80% in sensitivity has been reported by many authors using a planar acquisition. Using higher activities (7 to 10 mCi) associated with SPECT acquisition, the sensitivity would probably be increased. Whole body scanning is very useful in the evaluation of extra-thoracic locations.

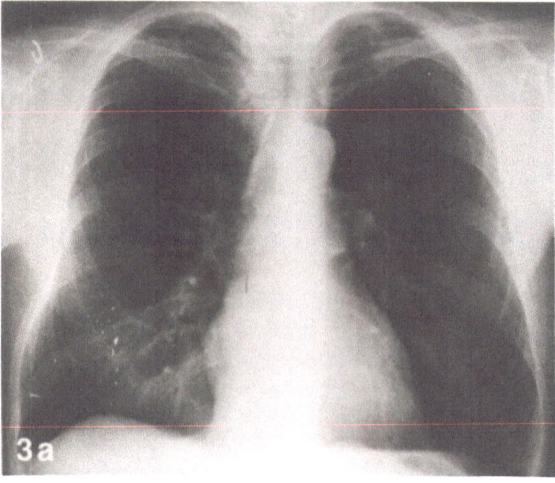
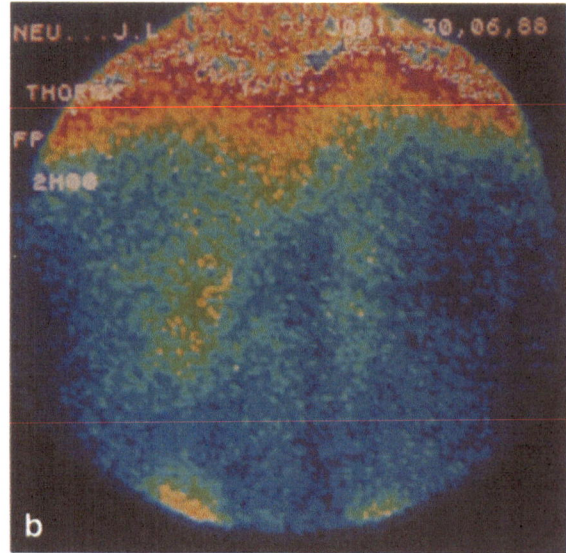

Fig. 3 a, b. Adenocarcinoma of the left lower lobe revealed by a symptomatic brain metastasis. This 56-year-old man had no respiratory symptoms and a normal chest roentgenogram **a.** Fiberoptic bronchoscopy showed a small tumor localized in the left lower lobe bronchus. J001 scintigraphy (posterior view) shows a high fixation in the area of the left lower lobe **b**

Gallium is not specific. Some authors reported a 91% positive predictive value for primary carcinoma of the lung. However the negative predictive value was only 76%. Due to its lack of specificity, the number of gallium scans decreased. Some authors now propose to improve the image quality of gallium scans by increasing the radionuclide activity in patients with proven tumors and using SPECT acquisition. Studies are in progress.

Macrophage scintigraphy

Despite improved resolution with new imaging techniques, the detection of tumor masses less than 1 cm in diameter remains difficult. A possible strategy could be the imaging of tumors via their associated macrophage population. The macrophage content of spontaneous metastases has been demonstrated to decrease rapidly during growth, reaching uniformly low levels by the time the metastases are 0.5 mm in diameter [19]. Immunomodulators of bacterial origin such as muramyl-dipeptide (MDP) or lipopolysaccharide (LPS) are able to bind to macrophages, thus activating them to a degree at which they become cytotoxic to cancer cells. However, both lack of specificity and low affinity limit the effectiveness of these agents for in vivo macrophage targeting.

These limitations for clinical use have led to the development of an approach based on macrophage imaging by J001X scintigraphy. J001X is a fully characterized 34 kDa acylated poly [1,3] galactoside isolated from Klebsiella membrane proteoglycans that is able to recognize macrophages selectively both in vitro and in vivo. Due to its amphiphatic properties, technetium-99m radiolabeled J001X is absorbed through the respiratory tract after aerosol administration. In these conditions, J001X rapidly diffuses in the blood, lymph and extracellular spaces. Kidney clearance of unbound J001X molecules occurs within 4 hours after administration. Images are obtained within 3 to 5 hours after inhalation.

Patients inhale the radiolabeled J001X preparation as an aerosol using an ultrasound TV 6000 inhaler. Aerosolization is always limited to 15 min to prevent any degradation of the tracer. To avoid false positive results resulting from skin contamination, patients wear gloves and clothes that are changed after inhalation and before each scintigraphy. Three and five hours after inhalation, anterior and posterior images are recorded.

The scintigraphic images are interpreted after digitized contrast enhancement by scaling the maximum of intensity to a lower value than the maximum count. The scintigraphy is considered normal when no activity is detectable in the lung, hilar regions or mediastinum 5 hours after inhalation. The radio-active J001X concentration in abnormal fixing areas is evaluated by an uptake index comparing the mean count in these areas to the non-specific vascular mean count in the shoulder area.

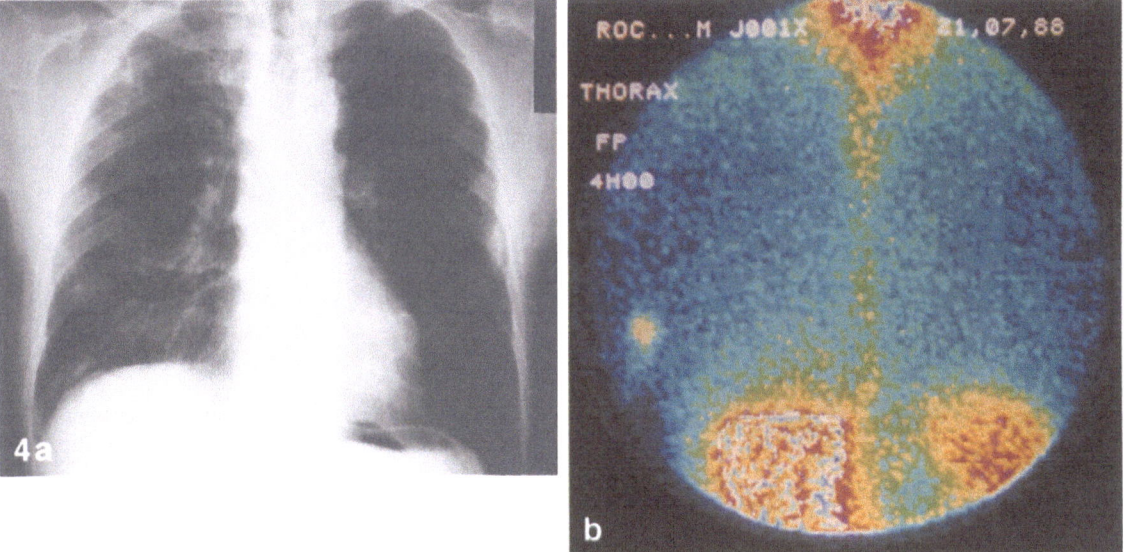

Fig. 4 a, b. Large cell carcinoma of the right upper lobe. **a** A posteroanterior roentgenogram of this 65-year-old man reveals a peripheral tumor of the right upper lobe with enlargement of the mediastinum due to metastatic lymph nodes. J001 scintigraphy (posterior view) shows a left axillary fixation corresponding to an histologically proved metastatic lymph node **b**

J001X scintigraphy was performed prior to therapy in 15 patients with lung cancer (figs. 3, 4). In 8 patients, positive abnormal fixing areas were found: mediastinal lymph nodes and hilar tumors (7 patients), metastatic proved axillary node (1 patient) and skin metastases (1 patient). In 2 patients, the positive mediastinal lymph nodes were 6 to 8 mm in diameter at the time of surgery. This study demonstrated that imaging could be achieved for tumor masses in the hilum corresponding either to the primary or contiguous lymph node involvement [20].

The purpose of a second study was to evaluate the ability of J001X scintigraphy to locate the extent of lymph node involvement in mediastinal and extra-thoracic areas [21]. Two groups of non-small cell lung cancers were studied. One group consisted of 6 peripheral tumors and the other consisted of 7 surgically confirmed non-small cell lung cancers with involvement of mediastinal lymph nodes and 5 inoperable non-small cell lung cancers with supraclavicular, axillary and mediastinal lymph nodes and metastases. In the first group, a fixation in the area of the tumor was observed in one patient. In the second group, 8 patients exhibited fixations both in the tumor and hilar lymph node areas in the supraclavicular area and axillary areas. These results confirmed that J001X scintigraphy is of value for the scintigraphic imaging of lung cancer. The observed fixations of J001X probably indicated the associated tumor lymph nodes

rather than the primary tumor. Among the metastatic lymph nodes, a high fixation was especially observed in the final nodes affected.

Further studies are necessary to define the clinical value of macrophage scintigraphy in lung tumors. Lack of specificity prevents its use for staging lung cancer. Macrophage scintigraphy could be valuable to detect residual or recurrent tumor tissue and thus appears to be complementary to immunoscintigraphy using MAbs.

SMS and MIBG scintigraphy

MIBG scintigraphy

Meta-iodobenzylguanidine (MIBG) is a marker of monoamine uptake in tissues and in tumors.

It is labeled with iodine-131 (^{131}I MIBG) or iodine-123 (^{123}I MIBG) (see chapter "Physical and technical bases", paragraph "Radiopharmaceuticals"). The injected activity is 37 MBq for ^{131}I MIBG and 130 MBq for ^{123}I MIBG. The scintigraphy is performed 24 and 48 hours after ^{131}I MIBG and 6 and 24 hours after ^{123}I MIBG (see chapter "Practical notions for carring out nuclear medicine examination"). The advantage of ^{123}I MIBG is the low radiation dose and the optimal physical detection properties (see chapter "Physical and technical bases").

Potentially MIBG could be used as a marker of pulmonary endothelial cells. It was shown in animals

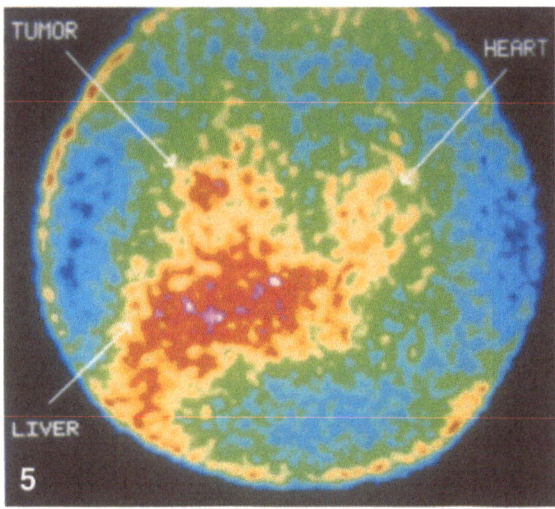

Fig. 5. Anterior view of the thorax 48 hours after ^{131}I-MIBG injection in a patient with a carcinoid tumor in the right lung. The concentration of MIBG is visible in the liver, heart and tumor

that MIBG uptake, as other amine uptakes, reflects cell metabolism [22]. However applications in human pathology have not yet been developed.

MIBG is principally a tumor marker: it is specifically taken up by tumors developed from the APUD (Amine Precursor Uptake and Decarboxylation) system: pheochromocytoma, neuroblastoma, medullary thyroid carcinoma and carcinoid tumor. Uptake is constant in the first two tumors [23-25], and about 25% in the medullary thyroid cancer [26]. Uptake was reported in 48 of 82 patients with carcinoid tumor, but in only 1 of 9 patients with a bronchial carcinoid tumor [27]. We found one positive case among five patients with thoracic carcinoid tumor (fig. 5).

SMS scintigraphy

Somatostatin is a hypothalamic tetradecapeptide, discovered 20 years ago. Initially known as a growth hormone secretion inhibiting factor, it proved to be an ubiquitous substance, synthesized in many organs with strong biological actions: endocrine and exocrine secretion inhibition, cell proliferation inhibition, gastro-intestinal mobility and regulation of vasomotility regulation. These actions involve binding to specific receptors in the target organs. These receptors are present in a number of tumors, specially APUD tumors such as small cell lung carcinoma. Stable somatostatin analogs have been synthesized: the octreopeptide Phe - Lys - Phe - Trp - Lys - Thr - Lys - Thr (SMS 201-995 Sandoz*) and the Tyr3 substituted octreopeptide (SMS 204-090 Sandoz*), radiolabeled with ^{123}I or [111]In (see Chapter "Physical and technical bases"). These radiolabeled analogs have the same affinity as somatostatin for receptors and specifically bind to tumor receptors.

Interesting preliminary scintigraphic results have been obtained in various tumors and specially in the small cell lung carcinoma. In five of eight patients with small cell lung carcinoma it was possible to visualize the tumor by [123]I - tyr 3 - octreotide scintigraphy. Unexpected metastases were found in two patients [28]. The value of this method is to provide specific topographic data on tumor localization, local and general extension, functional data on the presence of somatostatin receptors, which is important when considering treatment by somatostatin analogs, and dosimetric data with a view to treatment by metabolic irradiation.

References

1. Stein R, Goldenberg DM (1991) Prospect for the management of non-small-cell carcinoma of the lung with monoclonal antibodies. Chest 99 : 1466-1476
2. Kohler G, Milstein C (1975) Continuous cultures of fused cells secreting antibody of predefined specificity. Nature 256 : 495-497
3. De Land FH (1989) A perspective of monoclonal antibodies : past, present and future. Sem Nucl Med 19 : 158-165
4. Zuckier LS, Rodriguez LD, Scharff MD (1989) Immunologic and pharmacologic concepts of monoclonal antibodies. Sem Nucl Med 19 : 166-186
5. Bogard WC, Dean RT, Deo Y, Fuchs R, Mattis JA, McLean AA, Berger HJ (1989) Practical considerations in the production, purification, and formulation of monoclonal antibodies for immunoscintigraphy and immunotherapy. Sem Nucl Med 19 : 202-220

6. Goldenberg DM (1976) Oncofetal and other tumor-associated antigens of the human digestive system. Curr Top Pathol 63 : 239-242

7. Leitha T, Walter R, Schlick W, Dudczak R (1991) 99mTc-anti-CEA radioimmunoscintigraphy of lung adenocarcinoma. Chest 99 : 14-19

8. Poste G, Fidler IJ (1980) The pathogenesis of cancer metastases. Nature 283 : 139-145

9. Schlom J, Weeks MO (1985) Potential clinical utility of monoclonal antibodies in the management of human carcinomas. In : Devita VT, hellman S, Rosenberg SA (eds) Important advances in oncology. Lippincott, Philadelphia, pp. 170-192

10. Mansi L, Salvatore M, Del Vecchio S, Lapenta L (1986) Imaging of melanoma with T1C1 and monoclonal F (ab') 2. J Nucl Med 27 : 1022-1027

11. Horan Hand P, Colcher D, Salomon D, Ridge J, Noguchi P, Schlom J (1985) Influence of spatial configuration of carcinoma cell populations on the expression of a tumor associated glycoprotein. Cancer Res 45 : 833-839

12. Friedman S, Sullivan K, Salk D, Nelp WB, Griep RJ, Johnson DH, Blend MJ, Aye R, Suppers V, Abrams PG (1990) Staging non-small cell carcinoma of the lung using technetium-99m-labeled monoclonal antibodies. Hematology / Oncology Clin North Am 4 : 1069-1078

13. Bourguet P, Dazord L, Desrues B, Collet B, Ramee MP, Delaval P, Martin A, Logeais Y, Pelletier A, Toujas L (1990) Immunoscintigraphy of human lung squamous cell carcinoma using an iodine-131 labelled monoclonal antobody (Po66). Br J Cancer 61 : 230-234

14. Kwekkeboom DJ, Krenning EP, Bakker WH, Oei HY, Splinter TAW, Kho GS, Lamberts SWJ (1991) Radio-iodinated somatostatin analog scintigraphy in small-cell lung cancer. J Nucl Med 32 : 1845-1848

15. Kalofonos HP, Sivalopenko GB, Courtenay-Luck NS, Snook DE, Hooker GR, Winter R, McKenzie CG, Taylor-Papadimitriou JJ, Lavender PJ, Epenetos AA (1988) Antibody guided targeting of non-small cell lung cancer using 111In-labeled HMFG1 F (ab') 2 fragments. Cancer Res 48 : 1977-1984

16. Biggi A, Buccheri G, Ferrigno D, Viglietti A, Farinelli M C, Comino A, Leone A, Quaranta M, Taviani M (1991) Detection of suspected primary lung cancer by scintigraphy with indium-111-anti-carcinoembryonic antigen monoclonal antibodies (type F023C5). J Nucl Med 32 : 2064-2068

17. Larson SM (1985) Radiolabeled monoclonal antitumor antibodies in diagnosis and therapy. J Nucl Med 26 : 538-545

18. Courtenay-Luck N, Epenetos AA, Halnan KE, Hooker G, Hughes JMB, Krausz T, Lambert J, Lavender P, MacGregor WG, McKenzie CJ (1984). Antibody-guided irradiation of malignant lesions : three cases illustrating a new method of treatment. Lancet I : 1441-1443

19. Beckerman C, Hoffer P B, Bitran JD (1984) The role of Gallium-67 in the Clinical Evaluation of Cancer. Semin Nucl Med 4 : 296-323

20. Bugelski PJ, Corwin SP, North SM, Kirsh RL, Nicolson GL, Poste G (1987) Macrophage content of spontaneous metastases at different stages of growth. Cancer Res 47 : 4141-4145

21. Diot P, Le Pape A, Zaffreya S, Normier G, Dussourd D'Interland L, Binz H, Baulieu JL, Lemarié E (1989) Scintigraphy with a Klebsiella Membrane Glycopeptide (KMG) for the imaging of lung cancer : from the model of radio-induced carcinogenesis in baboons to human pathology. Am Rev Respir Dis 139 : A 216

22. Lemarié E, Diot P, Baulieu JL, Pascal S, Normier G, Binz H, Le Pape A (1990) Scintigraphy with D25, a klebsiella membrane glycopeptide, for the detection of lymph node metastases in lung cancer. Am Rev Respir Dis 4 : A57

23. Slosman DO, Morel DR, Mo Costabella PM, Donath A (1988) Lung uptake of 131I-metaiodobenzylguanidine in sheep. An in vivo measurement of pulmonary metabolic function. Eur J Nucl Med 14 : 65-70

24. Shapiro B, Copp JE, Sisson JC, Eyre PL, Wallis J, Beierwaltes WH (1985). Iodine-131 metaiodobenzylguanidine for the locating of suspected pheochromocytoma : experience in 400 cases. J Nucl Med 26 : 576-585

25. Shapiro B, Sisson J, Kalff V, Glowniack J, Satterley W, Glazer G, FrancisI, Bowers R, Thompson N, Orringer M (1984) The location of middle mediastinal pheochromocytomas. J Thor Cardiovascular Surg 87 : 814-820

26. Lumbroso J, Guermazi F, Hartmann O, Coornaert S, Raharison Y, Lemerle J, Parmentier C (1988) Sensitivity and specificity of meta-iodobenzylguanidine (MIBG) scintigraphy in the evaluation of neuroblastoma : analysis of 115 cases. Bull Cancer 75 : 97-106

27. Baulieu JL, Guilloteau D, Delisle MJ, Perdrisot R, Gardet P, Delepine N, Baulieu F, Dupont JL, Coutris G, Calmettes C (1987). Radioiodinated metaiodobenzylguanidine uptake in medullary thyroid cancer (MTC). A French cooperative study. Cancer 60 : 2189-2194

28. Hanson MW, Feldman JM, Blinder RA, Moore JO, Coleman RE (1989). Carcinoid tumors : iodine-131 MIBG scintigraphy. Radiology 172 : 699-703

Infectious diseases

A Moisan and ML Quinquenel

Detection of infectious sites constitutes a daily clinical problem. Generally, the diagnosis of infection is made by the association of a good physical examination, some laboratory tests and radiographic techniques. In some precise cases, scintigraphic techniques can be useful in order to reveal the localization of the infectious lesions rapidly. Most of these techniques are not very infection specific.

Over the last decades, experimental and clinical trials have been performed in order to find suitable radio-active agents and several scintigraphic methods have been proposed. Five main isotopic investigations are of value in infectious lung diseases. These are:

– gallium-67 scintigraphy;
– indium-111 labeled autologous granulocyte scintigraphy;
– technetium-99m HMPAO labeled leukocyte scintigraphy;
– labeled monoclonal antigranulocyte antibody scintigraphy;
– human nonspecific polyclonal immunoglobulin scintigraphy.

Methods

Gallium-67 scintigraphy (^{67}Ga)

Because of its concentration in inflammatory tissues, ^{67}Ga uptake is not specific and can be observed in many inflammatory processes (e.g. malignancy, sarcoidosis, pneumoconiosis, recent surgical wounds, etc) and many infectious diseases (e.g. tuberculosis, bacterial, viral or parasitic infections).

Patients' scans are performed 6 hours (T6) and possibly 24 hours (T24), 48 hours (T48) and 72 hours (T72) post-injection of 100 MBq of ^{67}Ga citrate. A medium energy collimator is used set over the 185 and 300 KeV gamma photon peaks of ^{67}Ga. The liver, bone, bladder, heart and sometimes the spleen can be visualized at T6; activity is also detected in the lungs and other soft tissues, corresponding to blood pool radio-activity. At T24 gut activity appears, and disappears normally at T72 if gut transit is regular.

In cases of infectious lesion, focal uptake can sometimes be detected at T6 but in most cases abnormal uptake is detected only on the last scintigrams.

Labeled leukocyte scintigraphy

Migration of granulocytes towards bacterial infectious sites is a well-known phenomenon. Separation, labeling in vitro and reinjection of patient granulocytes or labeling in vivo through the injection of a radiolabeled murine monoclonal anti-granulocyte antibody have been proposed in order to visualize infectious lesions. The former technique is frequently used whereas the evaluation of the latter is still in progress.

In vitro labeling procedure

Separation of granulocytes from peripheral blood cells is performed by sedimentation and centrifugation on Ficoll-metrizoate gradient. 107 granulocytes are necessary to perform the examination, so labeled granulocyte scintigraphy cannot be carried out if there is neutropenia. Two radioisotopes are used: indium-111 [1-3] and technetium-99m [4-6].

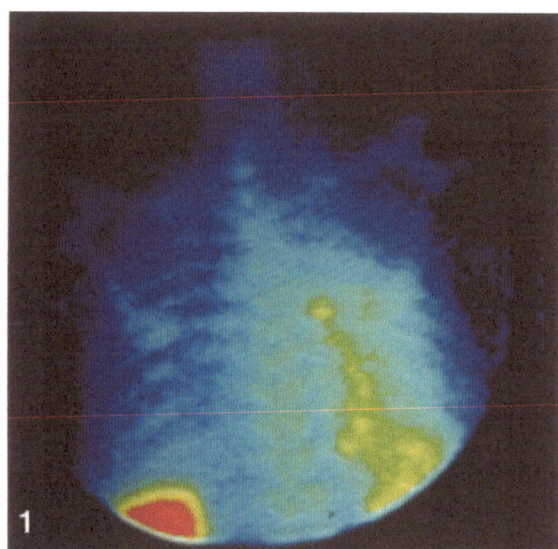

Fig. 1. Pulmonary localization of infection in a patient with septicemia (posterior view)

Indium-111 [1-3]

Indium-111 (T = 2.8 days) is used chelated with oxine; the resulting lipophilic complex penetrates the leukocyte membrane easily. Labeling is performed by addition of 10 to 15 MBq indium-111 to a white cell preparation rich in granulocytes (> 98%). In the final preparation, contamination by red blood cells remains less than 20%. Labeling efficiency averages 90% for indium-111 granulocytes. Intravenous injection contains 5 to 10 MBq indium-111 granulocytes.

Technetium-99m (^{99m}Tc)

Leukocyte labeling with [99m]Tc (T = 6 hours) is possible by different methods:

Sulphur colloid and stannous agent preparations have been tried but the low labeling yield, the high proportion of leakage of the radionuclide out of the cells in vitro and the great accumulation of radio-activity in the gut, have limited the development of these methods.

Hexamethylpropyleneamine-oxine (HMPAO) forms a lipophilic complex with ^{99m}Tc; this complex was first used for vascular brain imaging. [99m]Tc HMPAO easily penetrates blood cell membranes and remains intra-cellular better than the first compounds used [4]. Another advantage of ^{99m}Tc is the improvement in image quality with a lower radiation dose. The first studies to localize infectious diseases were performed in 1986 [4] and 1987 [5]. The labeling procedure can be performed on mixed leukocytes or on

a pure granulocyte preparation incubated with 99mTc HMPAO freshly prepared from a commercial kit. 200 to 300 MBq of ^{99m}Tc leukocytes are injected intravenously.

Scans are performed 3 hours and possibly 24 hours after intravenous injection. A gamma camera fitted with a parallel hole, medium energy collimator and 20% window set over the 173 and 247 KeV gamma photon peaks is used for In-111. For [99m]Tc a low energy collimator is used at 140 KeV photopeak with a window of 20%. A semi-quantitative study of the labeled cell uptake in the lungs is carried out with the data processing system. In bronchiectasis, sputum is also collected for 24 hours and radio-activity counted [3, 6].

Results

Granulocytes are localized in the spleen, liver and bone marrow, 2 to 3 hours post-injection and after their transit through the lungs.

There is a different behavior of radionuclides: urinary and biliary excretion may be observed 1 hour and 3 hours respectively after injection of ^{99m}Tc; there is no colonic or urinary elimination of indium-111.

In cases of infectious lesions, an increased focal uptake can be detected after injection for up to 24 hours for ^{99m}Tc and for up to 48 hours for indium-111.

In vivo labeling procedure [7, 8]

A murine monoclonal antibody against human granulocytes (AGAB) has been available since 1986. This antibody, an IgG (BW 250 / 183), binds to the carcinoembryonic antigen, a glycoprotein present on almost all human granulocytes. The cell binding is not cytotoxic.

Scans are performed 4-6 and 20-24 hours after intravenous injection of 500 MBq of the ^{99m}Tc labeled antibody. Scans are considered positive when a focally increased antibody accumulation occurs.

This method has not yet been evaluated for lung diseases in large series, but essentially in bone lesions. The procedure is very simple because cell separation and in vitro cell labeling are not necessary. Nearly all abscess lesions can be visualized only 4-6 hours after injection. Technetium-99m anti-granulocyte antibody scintigraphy is a promising method for detection of acute focal infectious lesions.

However the drawback of this method using a murine antibody, is the development of human-anti-mouse antibody (HAMA) sometimes with allergic reactions.

Tableau 1. Dosimetry

Vector injected dose X	Critical Organs	Absorbed dose per injected dose (mGy / X MBq)	Effective dose equivalent per injected dose (mSv / X MBq)
Gallium-67 citrate 100 MBq	Bones Gut Bone marrow	59 24 16	12
In-111 granulocytes 10-15 MBq	Spleen Liver Bone marrow	55 9,6 5,4	5,9
Technetium-99m HMPAO 10-15 MBq	Spleen Liver Bone marrow	31,4 4,8 3,7	3,3
Technetium-99m AGAB BW 250/183 500 MBq	Kidney Bone marrow	16,8 11,4	10
Technetium-99m HIG 400 Mbq	Kidney Gut Bone marrow	21,2 17,5 3,1	16,8

Human non-specific polyclonal immunoglobulin scintigraphy [7, 9]

Since 1988 a new agent has been proposed for scintigraphic detection of foci of infection. The mechanism of labeled Human polyclonal IgG (HIG) accumulation in inflammation and infectious foci has not been completely elucidated; accumulation is probably caused by increased vascular permeability and retention of the radiolabeled protein in the extravascular space [9]. HIG labeled with indium-111 or ^{99m}Tc is administered intra-venously (indium-111 HIG: 30 MBq; ^{99m}Tc HIG: 400 MBq).

Scintigrams obtained at 6, 24, and 48 hours (only for indium-111), successfully reveal various foci of infection. However specificity is poor: in some studies focal localizations also occurred in patients with cancer, sterile inflammatory arthritis, hematoma and recent fractures. In Oyen's first study in febrile patients with severe granulocytopenia, indium-111 HIG scans seem to be of interest to detect inflammation in early stages, especially for chest infections [9].

Table 1 shows that the effective dose equivalent for ^{99m}Tc HMPAO scintigraphy is half that for indium-111 granulocyte scintigraphy; for ^{67}Ga scintigraphy and for ^{99m}Tc AGAB scintigraphy, the critical organ is the bone marrow. For HIG scintigraphy the critical organs are the kidneys.

Indications and perspectives of scintigraphy

In the lung, the specificity of infectious disease localization varies according to the different scintigraphic methods. Gallium-67 scintigraphy is no longer indicated in this situation, except in immunocompromised patients.

Labeled granulocyte scintigraphy is more specific of infectious diseases. Indications can be limited to the exploration of secondary infectious lesions in septicemic patients or to finding occult infectious foci in patients with fever of unknown origin. In this case sensitivity is relatively low. In patients with correctly treated infections and persistent fever, scintigraphy can be useful to detect another focal infection or to confirm the disappearance of known foci; thus another cause of fever must be sought in this case [10, 11].

Some clinical studies have been carried out in order to find a marker of inflammation in bronchiectasis and possibly an index of activity of this disease. Studies have been made with indium-111 labeled granulocytes [3] and with ^{99m}Tc HMPAO labeled leukocytes

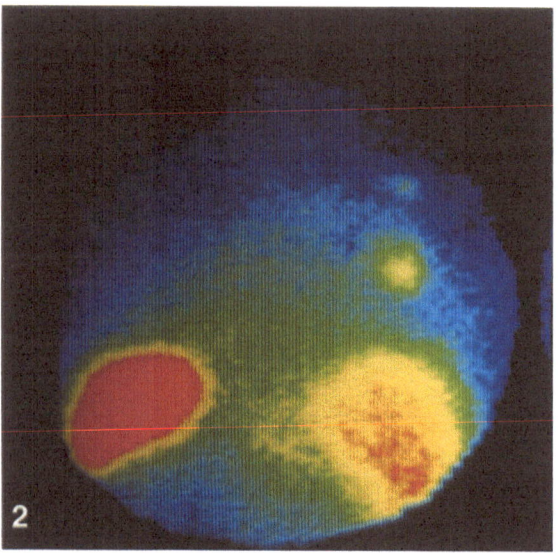

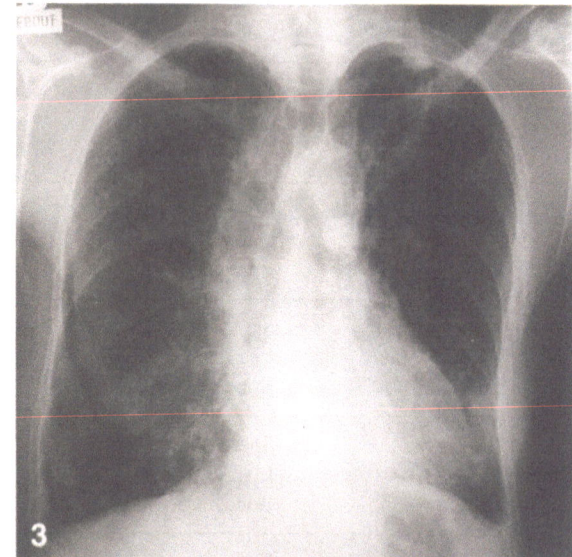

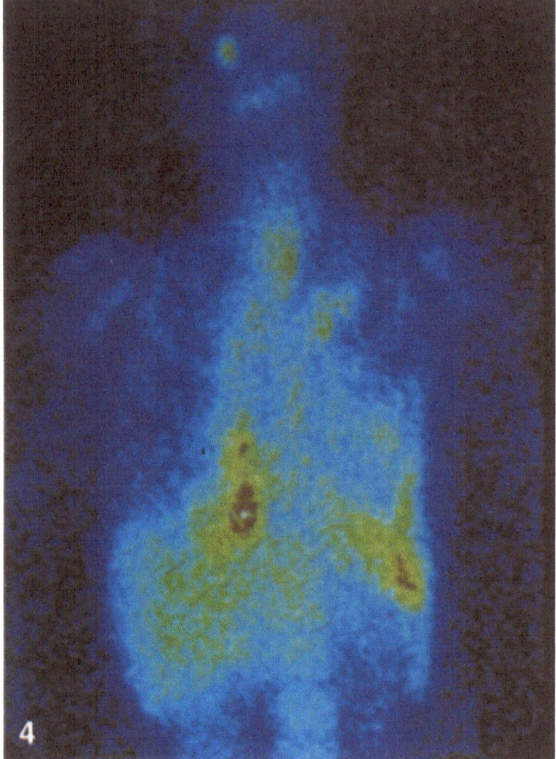

Fig. 2. Lung abscess in a patient with fever of unknown origin (posterior view)

Fig. 3. Chest X-ray in a patient with diffuse bronchiectasis

Fig. 4. ^{99m}Tc HMPAO labeled leukocyte scintigraphy in bronchiectasis (anterior view). Intense uptake in the right base of the lung 3 hours post-injection. Note also a focalized uptake in the right sinus which revealed purulent sinusitis

[6]. A good correlation has been found between scintigraphic activity and CT scan gravity score. These results need confirmation in large clinical trials.

Immunoscintigraphy is not performed in France at the present time. In some clinical studies it has not been proved to be reliable especially with the use of HIG [9]. However, this technique is time saving because it does not need in vitro cell preparation.

Conclusion

Bronchopulmonary or pleural infections do not generally require scintigraphic investigations, because chest X-ray and endoscopy or needle aspiration provide enough information for diagnosis or to guide treatment in most cases. Thus scintigraphy has very limited indications in pleuro-pulmonary infectious diseases and these rarely outweigh the cost of this relatively expensive examination.

References

1. Herry JY, Moisan A, Le Cloirec J (1986) Indium-111 autologous granulocytes in the diagnosis of abcess and in the assessment of inflammatory bowel disease. Nucl Med biol 13 : 183-190

2. Cook PS, Datz FL, Disbro MA, Alazraki NP, Taylor AT (1984) Pulmonary uptake in indium-111 leukocyte imaging : clinical significance in patients with suspected occult infections. Radiology 150 : 557-561

3. Liegaux JM, Moisan A, Delaval Ph, Desrues B, Bourguet P, Arnaud F, Kernec J (1989) Eur Respir J (suppl) 8 : 673

4. Peters AM, Osman S, Henderson BL, Kelly JD, Danpure HD, Hawker RJ, Hodgson HJ, Neirinekx RD, Lavender JP (1986) Clinical experience with ^{99m}Tc HMPAO for labeling leukocytes and imaging inflammation. Lancet 2 : 946-949

5. Mc Afee JG, Subramanian G, Gagne G, Scheider RF, Zapf-Longo C (1987) ^{99m}Tc-HMPAO for leukocyte labeling — experimental comparison with ^{111}In-oxine in dogs. Eur J Nucl Med 13 : 353-357

6. Quinquenel ML, Moisan A, Le Coz A, Desrues B, Devillers A, Briens E, Bourguet P, Delaval Ph (1992) ^{99m}Tc-HMPAO labeled leukocytes scintigraphy in bronchiectasis to detect inflammation. Am Rev Resp Dis 145 : A 774

7. Mc Afee JG, Gagne G, Subramanian G, and Schneider RF (1991) The localisation of indium-111-leukocytes, gallium-67 polyclonal IgG and other radioactive agents in acute focal inflammatory lesions. J Nucl Med 32 : 2126-2131

8. Hotze A, Briele B, Overbeck B, Kropp J, Gruenwald, Mekkawy MA, Von Smekal A, Moeller F, Biersack HJ (1992) Technetium-99m-labeled anti-granulocyte antibodies in suspected bone infectious. J Nucl Med 33 : 526-530

9. Oyen WJG, Claessens RAMJ, Van der Meer JWM, Strauss RHW, Corstens FHM (1992) Indium-111 labeled human non specific immunoglobulin G : a new radiopharmaceutical for imaging infectious and inflammatory foci. C I D 14 : 1110-1118

10. Mc Afee JG. Editorial (1990) What is the best method for imaging focal infections ? J Nucl Med 31 : 413-416

11. Williams JH (1991) Indium-111 labeled neutrophils for detecting lung injury. A perspective. Chest 99 : 1248-1251

Radionuclide imaging in pulmonary complications of Human Immunodeficiency Virus infection

J Cadranel, J Rosso, C Mayaud and M Meignan

The spectrum of pulmonary disorders associated with HIV infection includes both infectious and noninfectious diseases (table 1) [1,2]. In 1993, Pneumocystis carinii pneumonia (PCP) is still the most common HIV-related pulmonary infection in Europe and in the United States; other opportunistic pathogens are less frequent (although their relative incidence is increasing as the number of patients under PCP prophylaxis has risen and survival has been prolonged) [2]. Usual pathogens are also frequently found, particularly in Africa, and the frequency of tuberculosis is increasing elsewhere [2]. However, it must be kept in mind that the differential diagnosis of a suspected infection still includes several noninfectious complications (table 1) such as symptomatic pulmonary Kaposi sarcoma (KS) [1]. Furthermore, most of the patients have multiple infectious and noninfectious pulmonary complications simultaneously or alternately during the course of their HIV disease [1,2]. Since each pulmonary disorder requires a specific treatment, a definite diagnosis should be made each time a complication occurs and may often need repeated fiberoptic investigations [1,2]. Unfortunately, chest X-ray may be normal, clinical and radiological data are often non-specific and results obtained from pulmonary testing are neither specific nor sensitive in detecting pulmonary disease [1,2]. This emphasizes the need for new noninvasive procedures to limit the number of patients who really require exhaustive pulmonary diagnostic evaluation. In this context, two different radionuclides, gallium-67 citrate and technetium-99m diethylenetriamine pentaacetate (Tc-DTPA), have been used for assessment of the lungs of patients with HIV infection [3-5]. Gallium was used first as a means of detecting whether or not lung disease was present [6-18]. Tc-DTPA was then used, initially for research purposes, to study the permeability characteristics of the lung parenchyma, [19-22] but it has recently been considered more sensitive than gallium to detect PCP in HIV infected patients [23,24].

On the other hand, several teams have assessed the value of aerosolised pentacarinate therapy for the curative treatment and prophylaxis of PCP [5]. Radionuclide studies have also been used to define first the relative efficiency of nebulisers in pentamidine administration, and second possible optimization of this treatment [5]. The rationale and technical aspects of isotope applications for the development of aerosolised therapy are considered in a separate chapter of this book.

This chapter comprises two parts:
– gallium lung scanning in HIV infected patients;
– Tc-DTPA lung scanning in HIV infected patients.

Gallium lung scanning in HIV infected patients

Background

The mechanisms leading to gallium accumulation in regions of inflammation are unclear. After intravenous injection, gallium is believed to bind to transferrin and to migrate through the bloodstream to areas of

Table 1. Main pulmonary complications of HIV infection

Infections		
	Viruses	
		Cytomegalovirus
		Epstein-Barr virus (?)
		Human immunodeficiency virus (?)
	Bacteria	
		Pyogenic organism
		Nocardia asteroides, Rhodococcus equi
		Mycobacterium tuberculosis
		Mycobacterium avium complex
		Other Mycobacteria
	Fungi	
		Histoplasma capsulatum
		Coccidioides immitis
		Cryptococcus neoformans
		Aspergillus fumigatus
	Parasites	
		Pneumocystis carinii
		Toxoplasma gondii
		Cryptosporidia, Strongyloides stercoralis
Malignancies		
		Kaposi sarcoma
		Non-Hodgkin lymphoma
		Hodgkin lymphoma (?)
		Bronchial carcinoma (?)
Interstitial pneumonitis		
		Lymphocytic interstitial pneumonitis
		Nonspecific interstitial pneumonitis
Others (?)		
		Secondary alveolar proteinosis
		Drug-induced reactions
		Pulmonary embolism
		Bronchiolitis, emphysema

(?) Controversial results in the literature or diseases not included in the CDC definition of AIDS

inflammation where local increased permeability favors its extravasation and accumulation [5]. A small amount of gallium is taken up by inflammatory cells, but most remains extracellular in combination with lactoferrin and bacterial siderophore [5].

In general, the interpretation of the lung scan is based upon the intensity of gallium uptake in diseased areas and the amount of lung involved; some authors have suggested different scores to quantify the intensity of gallium uptake [5]. It may also be interesting to evaluate both the extra-pulmonary (mediastinal) and extra-thoracic (liver, spleen, lymph nodes) gallium uptake (see below) [3,5]. The appropriate interpretation of gallium lung scans, which is a matter of debate, has been extensively reviewed in Chapter "Principles of the imaging process and analysis of images".

Since the normal lung is not gallium avid, gallium scan was helpful in evaluating the presence and/or severity of inflammation arising from several infectious and noninfectious pulmonary disorders before AIDS [5]. It is worth mentioning that no specific caution has to be taken when using gallium scan in HIV infected patients apart from possible needle stick occurring in health workers during intravenous gallium injection.

Results of gallium lung scanning in AIDS patients with suspected pneumocystis carinii pneumonia

Specificity and sensitivity

Several case reports and a few clinical studies concerning 10 to 100 patients suggest a potential diagnostic role for gallium lung scans in AIDS patients

Table 2. Sensitivity and specificity of gallium scan for the diagnosis of Pneumocystis carinii pneumonia

Author	N° PCP/ N° Patients	Specificity (%)*	Sensitivity (%)
Coleman	11/21	92	100
Barron	18/37	94	94
Woolfenden	20/46	78	95
Folmer	5/15	83	100
Bitran	15/32	100	100
Tuazon	8/8	100	100
Kramer	29/86	83	97
Rosso	27/100	89	81

PCP: Pneumocystis carinii pneumonia. *Only intense gallium uptake was considered positive to define the specificity

with possible PCP, especially when chest radiograph and/or arterial blood gas results are normal or equivocal (table 2) [6-18].

The sensitivity of gallium lung scans for the diagnosis of PCP has been shown to be 81 to 100% [10-12, 14, 16-18, 24]. The differences in the sensitivity reported in the literature depend on many factors. Low sensitivity may be due to the administration of specific therapy before gallium lung scan evaluation, the absence of clinical symptoms (cough, fever, dyspnea) and the normality of the chest X-ray at presentation. In all studies, however, the sensitivity of gallium lung scans is better than that of chest X-rays, results of pulmonary function tests (PFTs) or arterial blood gas levels.

Gallium specificity for PCP detection is 78 to 100% (table 2) [10-12, 14, 16-18, 24]. This specificity depends primarily on the proportion of patients included in the studies who did not have PCP. In fact, in the different studies 25 to 70% of the patients had pulmonary infections other than PCP or noninfectious HIV-related pulmonary complications [10-12, 14, 16-18, 24] and all non-PCP infections may be at the origin of lung gallium uptake (table 3). Although some noninfectious HIV-related complications may also be linked to mild to moderate lung gallium uptake, it should be pointed out that in the different series of the literature, pulmonary KS in the absence of superimposed infection has never been associated per se with significant lung gallium uptake [16,18,24].

To increase gallium lung scan specificity for detection of PCP, some authors have emphasized the value of grading gallium uptake rather than simply describing a scan as being positive or negative [11, 16, 17]. There was a statistically significant greater incidence of lung uptake in scans associated with PCP than in those associated with other diagnoses; the specificity of gallium scan increased up to 95% when only scans with lung uptake more intense than that of the liver were considered as being positive for PCP [16]. Consideration of the distribution of gallium uptake may also increase the specificity of the scan for PCP. In the Kramer et al series, the positive predictive value of gallium scan for PCP with any intrapulmonary uptake was 62%; in contrast, it was increased to 72% and to 87% respectively when either simple diffuse uptake or heterogeneous and diffuse uptake were considered as being positive [16]. Finally, Baron et al found that the specificity of positive gallium also increased from 74% to 85% when patients with only normal or equivocal chest X-rays were taken into account [12].

Although gallium is notoriously nonspecific, it appears that in a symptomatic HIV seropositive patient with normal chest X-ray, a diffuse grade 3 or 4 gallium lung uptake has diagnostic value for PCP. Nevertheless, less prominent diffuse or focal gallium uptake should still lead to diagnostic discussion since even a minimal uptake is often associated with many AIDS-related infections or noninfectious pulmonary complications —except KS— requiring specific therapy (see below).

Value of gallium scanning follow-up after therapy for PCP

As suggested by the conflicting results of a small series, it is not clear whether an abnormal gallium scan following therapy simply represents pulmonary

Table 3. Patterns of pulmonary uptake of gallium citrate

No uptake
Kaposi sarcoma
Reactive lymphadenopathy
Suppressive lymphocyte alveolitis
Focal uptake
Intrathoracic/extrathoracic lymph nodes
Lymphoma
Mycobacterium avium complex
Mycobacterium tuberculosis
Cryptococcus neoformans
Intraparenchymal
Bacterial pneumonia
Lymphoma
Mycobacterium tuberculosis
Cryptococcus neoformans
Diffuse uptake
Mild to moderate
Cytomegalovirus
Mycobacterium tuberculosis
Cryptococcus neoformans
Cytolytic lymphocytes alveolitis
Lymphocytic interstitial pneumonitis
Nonspecific interstitial pneumonitis
Intense
Pneumocytis carinii pneumonia

inflammation or the persistence of active Pneumocystis carinii infection which should require prolonged therapy [10,11]. However, it is obvious that gallium uptake is lowered in patients showing favorable outcome under PCP therapy [10, 11].

Mechanism of gallium uptake in PCP

The reason for abnormal accumulation of gallium uptake in PCP is unclear. It may be related to the uptake of gallium by specific immune and inflammatory cells or to the leaking of protein-bound gallium from the inflamed vascular space [5]. Indeed, it is well known that diffuse epithelial injury is the main histological characteristic of human PCP [2]. In addition, it has been shown that experimental PCP results in pulmonary edema associated with abnormal gallium uptake with no increase in inflammatory cell infiltration and gallium accumulation within these inflammatory cells [3]. It has also been demonstrated in patients with PCP that the clearance of Tc-DTPA

from the lungs is raised and should be an early marker of PCP preceding abnormality of gallium scan (see below) [19-21].

Results of gallium lung scanning in AIDS patients free from pneumocystis carinii pneumonia

The frequency and specific pattern of abnormal gallium lung scans in patients with AIDS-related diseases other than PCP have not been well established [3]. Although PCP may be distinguished by intense diffuse gallium uptake, less intense uptake may also be related both to other pulmonary infections and noninfectious pulmonary complications. Important data have already been accumulated regarding the gallium pattern in AIDS-related pulmonary disorders other than PCP (table 3).

Results of gallium scan in non-PCP infections

Several authors have reported results of gallium lung scans in clinical settings of infectious pulmonary complications related to AIDS. If we consider the description of some case reports, CMV pneumonia results usually in mild-to-moderate diffuse lung gallium uptake [10, 12, 16, 24]; gallium scans may also show focal uptake or may be normal. In fact, in the absence of precise criteria for the definition of CMV pneumonia in AIDS, it is difficult to determine the role of gallium lung scans in the diagnosis of CMV pneumonia in such patients. In contrast, it is clear that fungallium infections may cause intense focal uptake or less intense diffuse patterns [10, 12, 16, 24].

Bacterial processes usually cause focal lung gallium uptake [16]; perihilar focal uptake has also been shown in one HIV seropositive patient with L. pneumophila pneumonia [16]. In tuberculosis, focal gallium uptake in AIDS and non-AIDS patients has been reported [13,24]; false negative results have however been found in both situations [13,15]. Atypical Mycobacterium avium intra-cellulare (MAIC) infection has been associated with minimal diffuse or patchy gallium uptake [10,15,18]. Nevertheless, more commonly mycobacteria infections result in focal gallium uptake within intrathoracic lymph nodes, often undetected by radiographic chest images [13, 16, 24]. Gallium can also disclose mycobacterial infections of extra-thoracic lymph nodes and bone marrow, often in clinically normal sites (see below)

Results of gallium scan in HIV-associated lymphoid processes

Lymphomas within or without the context of AIDS result in positive gallium uptake by the organs involved, e.g. mediastinal lymph nodes [3]. Such lymph node uptake cannot be distinguished from that observed in cases of mycobacterial infection without biopsy.

Other HIV-associated lymphoid processes i.e. lymphocytic interstitial pneumonitis (LIP) or non-specific interstitial pneumonitis (NSIP) may also be responsible for lung gallium uptake [18, 24-26]. These noninfectious pulmonary complications cannot be differentiated from PCP by clinical symptoms or pulmonary function tests, particularly in patients with normal chest X-ray. However, gallium lung scan in LIP and NSIP shows either more focal or less intense uptake than in PCP [18, 24].

Results of gallium scan in pulmonary Kaposi sarcoma

Unlike pulmonary infections or lymphoid processes in HIV seropositive patients, lung Kaposi sarcoma does not seem to be gallium-avid [1, 5]. In an AIDS patient with or without previously diagnosed cutaneous KS, the presence of interstitial and nodular changes on chest X-ray that do not label with gallium strongly suggest pulmonary KS [1, 5]. On the other hand, the presence of focal gallium uptake in the lungs or mediastinal lymph nodes of such a patient with KS is highly suggestive of concomitant infection and/or lymphoma [16,24].

Recently, after intravenous injection of Tc-pertechnetate (a radionuclide that concentrates in vascular lesions), focal uptake has been found in KS lesions that were clinically latent [5]. The specificity of this finding, however, has not yet been evaluated. The role of another radionuclide, thallium-201, has also been studied but still requires further investigation [1].

Comparison between gallium and indium-111-labeled autologous leukocyte lung scans

Labeled leukocytes have been used in AIDS to a lesser extent than gallium scanning. It has been found that gallium was more sensitive than indium for diffuse pulmonary processes: uptake of indium (40%) is less than gallium (100%) in patients with known PCP [3]. In focal pulmonary bacterial infections, indium was more sensitive [3]; however, bacterial pneumonias do not require scintigraphic identification since they are usually diagnosed by physical examination and chest X-ray.

Value of whole body gallium scanning in pulmonary complications of HIV infection

When performing gallium scanning to diagnose lung disorders, it may be beneficial to scan the whole body for evidence of extra-pulmonary foci of disease unrecognized by clinical examination [1, 2, 5]. Indeed, it has been shown that HIV patients suffering from infectious or noninfectious HIV related pulmonary complications may also demonstrate unusually prominent abdominal labeling and/or labeling of peripheral lymph nodes [5, 18]. These whole body scanning patterns are usually attributable to opportunistic infections or lymphomas. Interestingly, KS and reactive lymphadenopathy do not label with gallium [5].

Although whole body gallium scanning resulted in detection of extra-thoracic sites of pulmonary disease, the specific predictive value of such abnormalities in the setting of AIDS is unknown [5]. However, the presence of such an extra-thoracic gallium uptake may help the physician to select the less invasive and more effective procedure, i.e. peripheral lymph node biopsy or pulmonary invasive procedure, in order to establish a specific diagnosis of pulmonary disease [5]. Nevertheless, some lymphomas have been detected while scanning with gallium for presumed PCP; conversely, asymptomatic PCPs have also been disclosed while staging lymphoma with gallium in AIDS patients [5].

Guidelines for the use of gallium lung scanning in HIV seropositive patients

There are several types of gallium uptake associated with AIDS-related pulmonary diseases (table 3). The best established types include negative uptake of gallium in KS and diffuse intense pulmonary gallium uptake in PCP [11, 16, 18]. CMV pneumonitis, pulmonary mycobacterial infection, early PCP as well as LIP and SNIP may be associated with less intense diffuse uptake [10, 12, 13, 15, 16, 18, 25, 26]. Focal accumulation of gallium in the mediastinal lymph nodes is suggestive of lymphoma or infection due to Mycobacteria or fungi [3, 13, 16, 24].

AIDS patients with obviously abnormal chest X-rays do not need gallium scintigraphy; the work-up should go directly to diagnostic procedures to obtain a definite diagnosis. However, in patients with known pulmonary KS and new symptoms or chest X-ray abnormalities, gallium scan is indicated to distinguish progressive KS from superimposed pulmonary infection.

The value of gallium imaging lies in guiding the subsequent work-up in symptomatic patients, with or at risk of HIV infection, whose chest radiographs are normal [16]:
– if the lung scan is negative, attention should be drawn outside the thorax;
– if there is parenchymal uptake —diffuse or focal— diagnostic procedures are indicated to identify pulmonary infection;
– if there is hilar or mediastinal node uptake, biopsy of lymph nodes, liver, or bone marrow is indicated, possibly after whole body gallium scanning.

However, even of there is a diffuse intense pulmonary gallium uptake suggestive of PCP, an abnormal gallium scan should be considered non-specific; it can help guide diagnostic procedures (BAL, TBB, TPB etc) toward the sites of gallium uptake [4, 5].

Tc-DTPA lung scanning in HIV infected patients

Background

In contrast to gallium, which is administered intravenously and then accumulates in the whole body, Tc-DTPA is delivered to the lungs by means of an aerosol, after which it spreads through the respiratory tract epithelium, then within the endothelium, and finally is cleared by the blood stream. Alveolar clearance of inhaled Tc-DTPA is directly related to the integrity of the alveolar barrier, and provides an index of pulmonary epithelial permeability to solutes [3].

Mathematical models to calculate Tc-DTPA clearance as well as technical considerations concerning the choice of nebulizer delivery systems are described in Chapter "Physiopathological bases". The clearance rate is usually expressed in terms of percentage of decrease in the radioactivity per minute measured by a gamma camera in a particular region of interest, i.e. part of or entire lung fields [3].

It must be remembered that clearance of Tc-DTPA is increased in a wide variety of acute or chronic pulmonary disorders not related to HIV-infection but also as a result of multiple factors including cigarette smoking, intravenous heroin use or lung distention and body position [3, 27]. In these situations, the practical value of this aerosol technique for diagnostic procedures has been underestimated and studies were initially undertaken to evaluate the permeability characteristics of the lung parenchyma during known intra-pulmonary processes such as cytotoxic lymphocytic alveolitis or PCP [19, 22]. Though the results of this technique are non-specific, it has been recently pointed out that there are no false-negative Tc-DTPA scans in PCP, implying that normal clearance would obviate the need for additional invasive diagnostic procedures [24].

A final remark should be added before the extensive use of Tc-DTPA scans as a screening method in HIV seropositive patients suspected of having infectious pulmonary disease. Indeed, since Tc-DTPA is delivered to the lungs as an aerosol and could be responsible for an irritative cough, all preventive measures must be taken to obviate the risks of nosocomial pulmonary infection (M. tuberculosis, Pneumocystis carini etc) affecting other immunocompromised patients and even health care workers.

Assessment of pulmonary epithelial permeability in pulmonary complications of HIV infection

Pulmonary epithelial permeability in HIV associated lymphocytic alveolitis

Lymphocytic alveolitis is frequently observed in HIV-infected patients with or without detectable lung infections or tumor processes [1]. Alveolar HIV-specific-cytolytic-CD8-T-lymphocytes are mainly found in patients at early stages of the disease and are gradually replaced by suppressive-CD8-T-cells during the course of the disease [1]. This cytolytic-lymphocytic alveolitis (CLA) is sometimes associated with clinical symptoms with or without interstitial pneumonitis on chest X-ray and PFT abnormalities; pulmonary histological findings in these patients frequently demonstrate the presence of LIP or NSIP [1, 22].

Meignan et al have shown that patients with CLA have an increase in Tc-DTPA pulmonary clearance when compared with those with a similar lymphocytic alveolitis but in the latter the alveolitis is mainly composed of suppressive cells [22]; in these cases the Tc-DPTA pulmonary clearance is indeed normal. In addition, they also demonstrated that the increased Tc-DTPA clearance correlated with the intensity of the CLA [22]. Finally, they showed a significant relationship between the intensity of the CLA and the reduction of both KCO and PaO2 in these patients [22]. Taken together, these results suggest that the CLA observed, as a part of the in vivo normal immune response of the body against HIV infection in the lung, may induce deleterious effects on the alveolocapillary barrier [22]. The actual mechanism involved to explain these deleterious effects could be the release of mediators (IL1, intracellular enzymes, free radicals, TNF etc, mediators known to be responsible for alveolar barrier alterations) by HIV protein bearing alveolar macrophages which have been shown in vitro to be the target cells of the cytolytic lymphocytes [22].

Pulmonary epithelial permeability in PCP

As alteration of the alveolar epithelial layer is a characteristic of PCP, it has been suggested that evaluation of Tc-DTPA clearance in the lungs may be helpful in detecting in vivo changes in alveolar capillary membrane permeability in seropositive patients suffering from PCP. In this context, several authors recently showed that PCP are associated with a rise in lung Tc-DTPA clearance [19-21,23] resulting from a characteristic change from the normal monoexponentiel Tc-DTPA clearance curve to a biphasic curve with a rapid clearance half-life as demonstrated by O'Doherty et al [21]. This increased permeability preceding abnormalities of chest X-ray and blood gases and even gallium uptake resolved after treatment of PCP [19, 21, 23]. It has thus been suggested that Tc-DTPA clearance might be a good means of selecting patients for bronchoscopic diagnosis of PCP but this requires further confirmation (fig. 1).

Comparison of gallium lung scan and Tc-DTPA clearance in pulmonary complications of HIV infection

Although previous short series addressed the question of the sensitivity of Tc-DTPA aerosol for the diagnosis of PCP, none of these studies compared the results obtained by both Tc-DTPA and gallium scanning for the detection of HIV-related pulmonary disorders.

More recently, Rosso et al compared the results obtained by these two radionuclide imaging methods in a large series of HIV patients [24]; indeed one hundred Tc-DTPA aerosols and gallium chest scans were performed in 88 symptomatic or asymptomatic patients infected with HIV presenting with normal chest X-ray or diffuse opacities (table 4). This study showed that Tc-DTPA scan was the most sensitive procedure for detecting pulmonary disorders related to HIV infection [24]. The sensitivity of a high clearance rate was 92% for infectious pulmonary complications (PCP and other pathogens) and 60% for non-infectious pulmonary complications (KS, cytolytic and suppressive alveolitis). As for arterial blood gases, chest X-ray and gallium scans, they had a sensitivity of 46%, 69% and 72% respectively in the detection of infectious diseases and 33%, 43% and 14% respectively in the detection of noninfectious disorders [24]. However, the sensitivity for the detection of PCP was similar when using both gallium scan (81%) or Tc-DTPA (85%) (table 4).

A 60% sensitivity of Tc-DTPA scan to detect noninfectious pulmonary complications appeared fairly good; however, Tc-DTPA scan compared to gallium scan was more sensitive. Nevertheless, this series mainly concerned patients with normal chest X-ray or diffuse pulmonary opacities; the sensitivity of these two procedures has not been evaluated for patients presenting hilar adenopathies or focal abnormalities on chest X-ray. This poor sensitivity was mainly due to the inclusion of a large group of

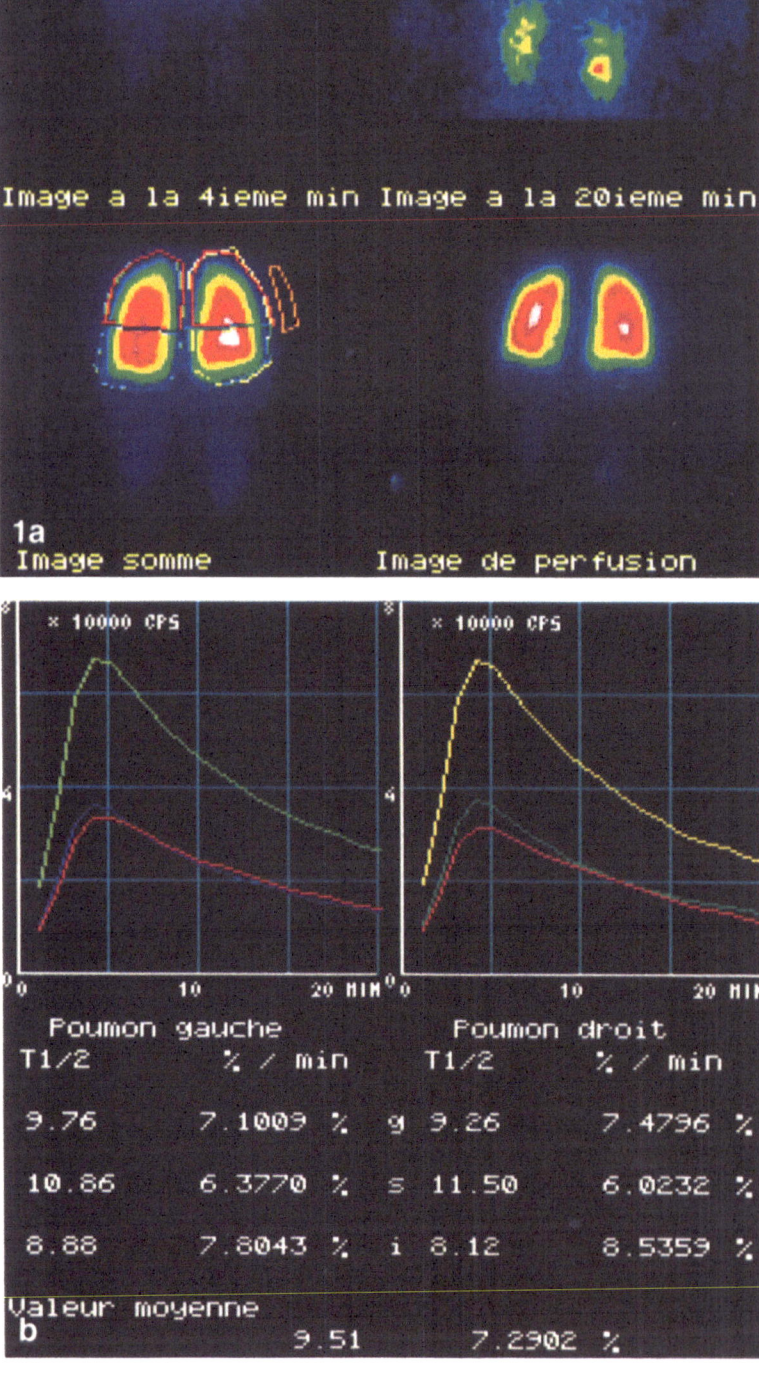

Fig. 1 a, b. HIV+ patient who had cough without fever. The chest X-ray and thoracic CT were normal. ^{99m}Tc-DTPA lung clearance was dramatically increased (**a, b**). Bronchoalveolar lavage demonstrated pneumocystis carinii

Table 4. Comparisons of Tc-DTPA and gallium scanning for the diagnosis of pulmonary complications of HIV infection, from [24]

	Positive gallium scan n (%)	DTPA clearance > 1.8% x min^{-1} n (%)	DTPA clearance > 4.5% x min^{-1} n (%)
Asymptomatic			
Nonsmokers (n=12)	0	0	0
Smokers (n=7)	0	5 (71)	1 (14)
Infections			
Pneumocystis Carinii (n=27)	22 (81)	27 (100)	23 (85)
Others (n=10)	7 (70)	6 (60)	0
Non infectious complications			
Kaposi sarcoma (n=7)	0	6 (86)	1 (14)
Cytotoxic alveolitis (n=17)	5 (29)	16 (94)	6 (35)
Suppressive alveolitis (n=13)	0	0	0

patients who had only suppressive lymphocytic alveolitis. However, if the patients with suppressive alveolitis were excluded, the sensitivity of Tc-DTPA scan improved to 92% while the sensitivity of gallium scan did not significantly increase.

More importantly, this high sensitivity means that a normal Tc-DTPA clearance rate virtually rules out pulmonary complications in HIV-seropositive patients. Also, Tc-DTPA scan appeared particularly helpful in this series for the detection of pulmonary disorders in patients with normal chest X-ray and arterial blood gases since Tc-DTPA clearance was accelerated in almost all of these patients except those with suppressive alveolitis only.

Unfortunately, the Tc-DTPA technique does lack specificity. A moderately increased clearance rate cannot help distinguish the various pulmonary disorders from each other nor those related to cigarette smoking (table 4). In this context, the authors proposed a cutoff value —more than 4.5% x min^{-1}— for a fast clearance rate which would be highly suggestive of PCP; a result higher than this cutoff value provides a sensitivity of 85% and a specificity of 87% for this diagnosis. It must be remembered, however, that these results should be taken with caution. First, they largely depend on the number of patients and the types of pulmonary disorders included. Second, some high clearance rates may be due to CLA and the drugs used to treat patients with PCP may cause pulmonary toxic reactions [5, 24]. Therefore, as for gallium scan, in the

case of abnormal Tc-DTPA scan, histologic diagnosis of PCP is needed before prescription of specific treatment.

Are there recommendations for the use of Tc-DTPA scanning in HIV seropositive patients?

In addition to its higher sensitivity demonstrated only by one group— several advantages in comparison with gallium imaging have been stressed. It is readily available, less expensive, rapidly performed and the results allow faster analysis [3, 14].

In view of these conclusions, modification of the diagnostic algorhythm has been proposed in non-smoker AIDS patients with fever and/or respiratory symptoms, based on gallium scan analysis [24, 25, 27]. When a non-smoker patient has a normal chest X-ray, Tc-DTPA aerosol scanning should be performed first if:

– the Tc-DTPA clearance is normal, then etiologic investigations should be directed to regions other than the chest;

– the Tc-DTPA clearance is accelerated, then a gallium scan may be indicated to guide the clinician toward an appropriate site for biopsy. When a patient has known pulmonary KS with abnormal chest X-ray, a gallium scan should be performed alone (see above).

Conclusion

The only way of identifying with certainty the cause of clinical and/or radiological respiratory disorders is based on direct diagnostic procedures such as induced sputum, fiberoptic bronchoscopy, thoracoscopy and sometimes open lung biopsy. However, the growing number of HIV-infected patients and the risks linked to some diagnostic procedures lead to selection of patients for whom the use of these invasive investigations is justified. Radionuclide tests appear very helpful in this selection.

In usual practice, the use of radionuclides is indicated in two clinical settings:

– in a patient with a new radiological abnormality due either to infection or KS determination, gallium scan could be of diagnostic value whether or not radionuclide uptake is observed;

– in a patient with an unexplained fever and/or respiratory symptoms associated with an apparently normal chest X-ray, the evaluation of the Tc-DTPA test could be worthwhile if subradiological diffuse parenchymal lesions are suspected; a positive result could then indicate the need for invasive investigations. It should be remembered that in such patients, other indirect diagnostic techniques have been suggested e.g. gallium, CT scan, DLCO evaluation and exercise test. As the sensitivity of these procedures is fairly high, the choice is based on reliability and availability at the site where the tests are performed.

References

1. White DA, Matthay RA (1989) Noninfectious pulmonary complications of infection with the human immunodeficiency virus. Am Rev Respir Dis 140 : 1763-1787
2. Murray JF, Mills J (1990) Pulmonary infectious complications of human immunodeficiency virus infection. Am Rev Respir Dis 141 : 1356-1372
3. Golden JA, Sollitto RA (1988) The radiology of pulmonary disease. Chest radiography, computed tomography and gallium scanning. In : White DA, Stover DE (eds) Pulmonary effects of AIDS. WB Saunders Company, Philadelphia, p 481
4. Ganz W, Serafini AN (1989) The diagnostic role of nuclear medicine in the acquired immunodeficiency syndrome. J Nucl Med 30 : 1935-1945
5. Kramer EL, Divgi CR (1991) Pulmonary applications of nuclear medicine. In : Naidich ND, Garay SM (eds) Imaging strategies in pulmonary disease. WB Saunders Company, Philadelphia, p 55
6. Liebman R, Ryo UY, Bekerman C, Pinsky SM (1982) Ga-67 scan of a homosexual man with Pneumcystis carinii pneumonia. Clin Nucl Med 7 : 480-481
7. Parthasarathy KL, Bakshi SP, Bender MA (1982) Radiogallium scan in P. carinii pneumonia. Clin Nucl Med 7 : 71-74
8. Levin M, Mc Leod R, Young Q et al (1983) Pneumocystis pneumonia : importance of gallium scan for early diagnosis and description of a new immunoproxydase technique to demonstrate Pneumocystis carinii. Am Rev Respir Dis 128 : 182-185
9. Moses, Baker SR, Seldin MF (1983) Diffuse pulmonar gallium accumulation with a normal chest radiogram in a homosexual man with Pneumocystis carinii pneumonia. A case record. Clin Nucl Med 8 : 608-609
10. Coleman DL, Hattner RS, Luce JM, Golden JA, Murray JF (1984) Correlation between gallium lung scans and fiberoptic bronchoscopy in patients with suspected Pneumocystis carinii pneumonia and the acquired immune deficiency syndrome. Am Rev Respir Dis 130 : 1166-1169
11. Tuazon CU, Delaney MD, Simon GL, Witorsch P, Varma VM (1985) Utility of gallium-67 scintigraphy and bronchial washings in the diagnosis and treatment of Pneumocystis carinii pneumonia in patients with acquired immunodeficiency syndrome. Am Rev Repir Dis 132 : 1087-1092
12. Barron TN, Birnbaum N, Shane L, Goldsmith SL, Rosen MJ (1985) Pneumocystis carinii pneumonia studied by gallium-67 scanning. Radiology 154 : 791-793
13. Bach MC, Bagwell SP, Masur H (1986) Utility of gallium imaging in the diagnosis of Mycobacterium aviu-mintracellulare infection in patients with the acquired immunodeficiency syndrome. Clin Nucl Med 11 : 175-177
14. Folmer SCR, Danner SA, Bakker AJ et al (1986) Gallium-67 lung scintigraphy in patients with acquired immunodeficiency syndrome. Eur J Respir Dis 68 : 313-318
15. Sharzynski JJ, Sherman W, Lee HK, Berger H (1987) Patchy uptake of gallium in the lungs of AIDS patients with atypical mycobacterial infection. Clin Nucl Med 12 : 507-509
16. Kramer J, Sanger JJ, Garay SM et al (1987) Gallium-67 scans of the chest in patients with acquired immunodeficiency syndrome. J Nucl Med 28 : 1107-1114
17. Bitran J, Beckerman C, Weinstein R, Bennett C, Ryo U, Pinsky S (1987) Patterns of gallium-67 scintigraphy in patients with acquired immunodeficiency syndrome and the AIDS related complex. J Nucl Med 28 : 1103-1106
18. Woolfenden JM, Carrasquillo JA, Larsen SM (1987) Acquired immunodeficiency syndrome : gallium-67 citrate imaging. Radiology 162 : 383-387
19. Mason GR, Duane GB, Mena I, Effros RM (1987) Accelerated solute clearance in Pneumocystis carinii pneumonia. Am Rev Respir Dis 135 : 884-868
20. Picard C, Meignan M, Rosso J, Cinotti L, Mayaud C, Revuz J (1987) 99mTc-DTPA aérosol and gallium scanning in acquired immune deficiency syndrome. Clin Nucl Med 12 : 501-506

21. O'Doherty MJ, Page CJ, Bradbeer CS et al (1989) The place of lung ^{99m}Tc-DTPA aérosol transfer in the investigation of lung infections in HIV-positive patients. Respir Med 83 : 395-401

22. Meignan M, Guillon JM, Denis M et al (1990) Increased epithelial permeability in HIV-infected patients with isolated cytotoxic T-lymphocytic alveolitis. Am Rev Respir Dis 141 : 1241-1248

23. Robinson DS, Cunningham DA, Dave S, Fleming J, Mitchell DM (1991) Diagnostic value of lung clearance of ^{99m}Tc-DTPA compared with other non-invasive investigations in Pneumocystis carinii pneumonia in AIDS. Thorax 46 : 722-726

24. Rosso J, Guillon JM, Parrot A et al (1992) Technecium-99m-DTPA aérosol and gallium-67 scanning in pulmonary complications of human immunodeficiency virus infection. J Nucl Med 33 : 81-87

25. Schiff RG, Kabat L, Kamani N (1987) Gallium scanning in lymphoid interstitial pneumonitis in children with AIDS. J Nucl Med 28 : 1915-1919

26. Zuckier LS, Ongseng F, Goldbarb CR (1988) Lymphocytic interstitial pneumonitis : a cause of pulmonary gallium-67 uptake in a child with acquired immunodeficiency syndrome. J Nucl Med 29 : 707-711

27. Stafianakis GN, Jabir AM, Beach et al (1989) Increased gallium-67 pulmonary activity in human immunodeficiency virus (HIV) positive non AIDS, non-ARC, non-IV drug abusers : correlation with tobacco smoking. J Nucl Med 29 : 829

Chronic obstructive pulmonary diseases

F Baulieu, S Coequyt and JJ Lafitte

Chronic obstructive pulmonary diseases (COPD) comprise several lung diseases which share the characteristics of obstruction of the airways and hypersecretion. The majority of patients have chronic bronchitis, chronic asthma and emphysema. Chronic bronchitis is an extremely common disease defined by the World Health Organization as "a persistent cough with excessive production of sputum for 3 or more months in the year for 3 successive years". Typically, the patient is a middle-aged heavy smoker with recurrent respiratory infections. Emphysema and chronic bronchitis usually occur together because they have common etiological factors, i.e. cigarette smoking and air pollution. Emphysema is described as a condition of the lungs characterized by an increase in the volume of the air spaces distal to the terminal bronchioles with destruction of alveolar tissue. Asthma is defined as variable airway obstruction. The changes in severity of airway narrowing can occur spontaneously or as a result of therapy. Complete remission usually occurs between attacks. In some chronic asthma patients, the airway obstruction is not reversed by bronchodilatator agents.

Mucociliary clearance

Mucociliary escalator

The respiratory system is exposed to external aggression due to environmental particles. Mucocilary clearance is a defense mechanism that is necessary to preserve the integrity of bronchopulmonary structures. Thus, in addition to cellular and biochemical defense mechanisms, lung protection is assured by mechanical processes to eliminate pathogenic agents. These mechanical processes depend on ventilation and moreover on ciliary beating and mucus production.

Mucus is an heterogenous liquid composed of two phases, "sol and gel". Mucus is produced permanently with successive periods of secretion and absorption. Its biochemical and rheological properties correspond to anatomical and physiological properties of the respiratory tract, from the alveoli to the trachea. Alveolar surfactant, which is produced by alveolar granulocytes (type II), travels along the tracheo-bronchial tree, mixing with mucus from submucosal glands and goblet cells of the surface epithelium.

Ciliary activity facilitates mucus transport. Approximately 200 cilia per cell have very well co-ordinated beating at a frequency of 10 to 20 Hertz. These cilia propel mucus at a few millimeters per minute. Velocity increases from the small peripheral bronchi to the central main bronchi.

Methods for the evaluation of mucociliary clearance

The available techniques to evaluate mucociliary function are the study of the physical and biochemical properties of mucus, ciliary activity on isolated cells and overall mucociliary activity.

A large number of biochemical components of mucus such as proteins, glycoproteins (alpha 1 antitrypsin, immunoglobulins A and G), and phospholipids have been identified and are titrable. Mucins have a role in rheologic properties. Some disorders have characteristic hydration levels. For

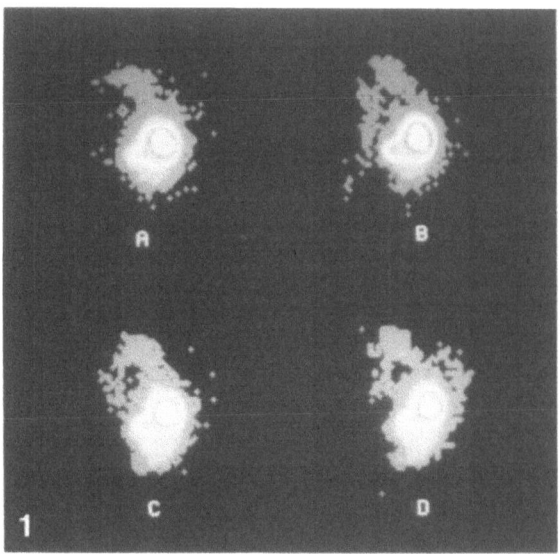

Fig. 1. Gastro-esophageal reflux (GER) and aspiration. *A* 3 min picture: GER; *B* 4 min picture: GER and right pulmonary aspiration; *C* 24 min picture: GER and right pulmonary aspiration; *D* 26 min picture: GER and bilateral pulmonary aspiration

example, cystic fibrosis mucus contains 85% water whereas the mucus of normal patients contains 95%. The rheological characteristics of the mucus, i.e. viscocity, ropiness, elasticity and adhesivity, which are related to the biochemical composition, are measurable in the bronchial secretions.

In order to study ciliary structure and their beating function, biopsy specimens or cytologic aspirations are sampled on nasal mucosa via a nasal speculum or on the bronchial epithelium during fiberoptic bronchoscopy examination. Samples are analysed with a light or electron microscope. Ciliary beating can also be evaluated with light microscopy, microcinema or stroboscopic measurement of frequency of ciliary beating.

Mucus velocity can be quantified using a radioactive or a radioopaque index to measure the speed of the moving index. Mucociliary clearance can be quantified using a radioactive tracer that is first deposited in large, proximal airways.

Mucociliary clearance study in clinical practice

Diagnostic value of mucociliary clearance study

The origin of recurrent bronchial infections or bronchiectasis is often difficult to determine. On the other hand, impairment of mucociliary clearance is often observed in chronic bronchopulmonary diseases. In fact, at an advanced stage, dyskinesia and ciliary immobility are not always diagnosed by mucociliary clearance study. In contrast, normal mucociliary clearance in a patient suffering from chronic bronchopulmonary disease can eliminate dyskinesia or a primary ciliary immobility syndrome [1]. Moreover, mucociliary clearance study represents only an instantaneous picture of clearance function and must take into account recent acute bronchial infections.

Evaluation of pharmacological agents on lung mucociliary clearance

The efficacy of mucolytic agents or expectorants is difficult to evaluate. Mucociliary clearance study has been proposed for this purpose. In fact, study results are conflicting. These differences may be explained by the various techniques that are used and the clinical variations between patients. Indeed an obstructive syndrome can modify the mucociliary clearance data obtained [2].

Gastro-esophageal scintigraphy

The association of gastro-esophageal reflux (GER) and recurrent pulmonary disease was first recognized in the late 19th century. Patients with atopic asthma, chronic lung disease of unknown origin have an increased incidence of GER. This pathology is common in children and can occur in adults.

The pulmonary disease is presumably due to aspiration of gastric content. Pulmonary disease associated with GER is not always the result of pulmonary aspiration. In asthmatic patients with GER, wheezing can be reproduced by an infusion of hydrochloric acid directly into the esophageus and would be a consequence of an eso-bronchic reflux. The event of reflux may induce bronchospasm and chronic asthmatic symptoms through reflex vagal mechanisms or recurrent aspiration.

Gastro-esophageal scintigraphy is a valuable technique for the detection of GER; it provides a non-invasive means for diagnosing pulmonary aspiration [3, 4].

Scintigraphic procedure

Scintigraphy is usually performed after a 12 hr fasting period. The patient swallows the tracer (^{99m}Tc sulfur colloid) mixed with some milk and then the rest of the unlabeled milk in order to clear the mouth and esophagus of any residual activity. The recording is made in the supine position from an anterior view and consists of 60 consecutive 1 min frames. Static pictures, in anterior, posterior and lateral views, are usually obtained at 1hr and 4 hrs.

The pictures are visualized first without and then with contrast enhancement, by lowering the upper threshold to about 30% of the maximal count rate. Enhancement of the computer images is necessary for vizualisation of pulmonary aspiration and minimal reflux. Pulmonary aspiration is characterized by a localized accumulation of activity in the lungs (fig. 1).

When a pulmonary area is detected, activity due to contamination must be carefully excluded in order to avoid misinterpretation.

Quantitative assessment is simply performed from the esophageal time activity curve of the first hour. GER can be quantified as the background corrected ratio of esophageal to initial gastric radioactivity [5].

In conclusion, dynamic scintigraphy is a simple technique for the demonstration of GER and aspiration. It remains the only technique for the visualization of pulmonary aspiration. The pulmonary aspiration, when demonstrable, should be considered as a possible cause or contributing factor of asthma.

References

1. Rühle KH, Köhler D, Fischer J, Matthhys H (1979) Measurement of mucociliairy clearance with ^{99m}Tc-target erythrocytes. Prog Resp Res 11 : 117-126
2. Mezey RJ, Cohn MA, Fernandez RJ. (1978) Mucociliary transport in allergic patients with antigen-induced bronchospasm. Am Rev Resp Dis 118 : 677-684
3. Boonyaprapa S, Alderson PO, Garkinkel DJ et al (1980) Detection of pulmonary aspiration in infants and children with respiratory disease : concise communication. J Nucl Med 21 : 314-318
4. Heyman S, Kirkpatrick JA, Winter HS et al (1979) An improved radionuclide method for the diagnosis of gastroesophageal reflux and aspiration in children (milk scan). Radiology 131 : 479-82
5. Baulieu F, Maurage C, Baulieu JL et al (1984) A quantitative approach to gastroesophageal reflux in children. Nucl Med Comm 5 : 689-695

Right-to-left shunt

JL Baulieu

A right-to-left shunt occurs when a part of the venous blood short-circuits the pulmonary alveoli and directly passes into the systemic circulation. Normally a part of mediastinal, portal, bronchial and myocardial venous blood flows into the left cavities resulting in a physiologic shunt, about 1 to 2% of the cardiac output. In pathologic conditions, much greater shunts may be encountered: extrapulmonary shunts due to congenital cardiac malformation, congenital or acquired pulmonary fistula, specially in liver cirrhosis, intra pulmonary atelectasis, acute edema or pneumopathy [1]. It is important to identify the right-to-left shunt because it is responsible for oxygenotherapy resistant hypoxemia. Shunt is often associated with other respiratory or circulatory disorders and often occurs in very debilitated patients. Thus, a specific and noninvasive diagnostic procedure is required.

The diagnosis of right-to-left shunt can be very simply made by ^{99m}Tc macroagregate or microsphere scintigraphy. The appearance of extrapulmonary activity in the brain and kidneys demonstrates the existence of a right-to-left shunt (fig. 1).

The localization of the shunt can be assessed by the analysis of the evolution of activity. The shunt corresponds to a zone of transient activity, constrasting with the stable activity due to normal capillary trapping. This analysis requires dynamic acquisition and can be automatically performed by the image processing called factor analysis. Factor analysis is capable of separating partially overlapping structures by automatically extracting factors with different temporal behaviour [2].

The quantitation of the shunt is classically performed using the equation [3]:

$$\frac{(\text{Total body count} - \text{total lung count}) \times 100}{\text{total body count}} = \% \text{ right-to-left shunt}$$

Total body count can be estimated from brain and kidney count by assuming that the brain and kidneys receive 38% of the cardiac output [2].

$$\text{Total body count} = \frac{(\text{brain count} + \text{background substracted kidney count})}{38} \times 100$$

The shunt can also be evaluated from the first pass activity curve in the pulmonary artery and in the shunt after ^{99m}Tc pertechnetate I.V. injection. Again, factor analysis is useful for automatically delineating pulmonary artery and shunt image. The area under the pulmonary artery and shunt curves are respectively proportional to flow. The percentage of pulmonary artery flow that goes to the shunt is a direct measure of the right-to-left shunt [2]. This method is appropriate when total body activity cannot be obtained. However, brain and kidney activity underestimates cardiac output in cases of renal insufficiency or brain hypoperfusion.

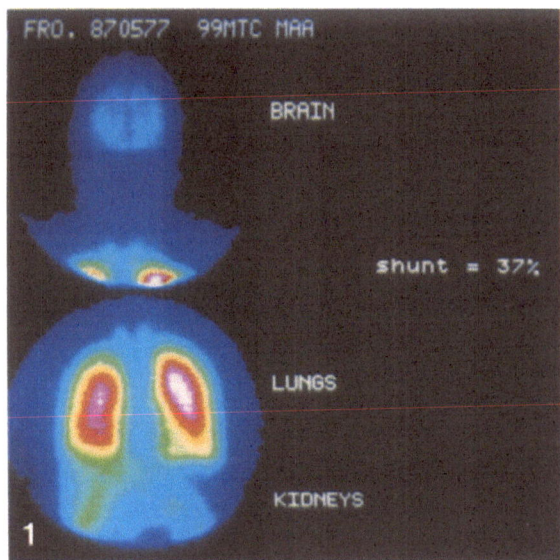

Fig. 1. Anterior view of the head and the thorax after ^{99m}Tc macroaggregate injection in a patient with a right-to-left pulmonary shunt. Note the extra-pulmonary activity in brain, liver and kidneys. The shunt flow was 37% of the cardiac output

References

1. Meyer P (1977) Physiologie Humaine 1, Flammarion, pp. 150-152
2. Villanueva-Meyer J, Marcus C, Thompson K, Philippe L, Mena I (1986) Diagnosis et quantification of pulmonary artériovenous malformation by factor analysis. Clin Nucl Med 11 : 88-91
3. Gates G, Orme H., Dore E (1971). Measurement cardiac shunting with technetium-labeled albumin aggregates. J Nucl Med 12 : 746-749

Nuclear Medicine and the pediatric lung

D Poncin, F Bonnin and B Bok

Nuclear Medicine has now gained acceptance as a useful, non-invasive and safe procedure in children [1-3]. Radionuclide investigations have been used to assess regional lung function and therefore can improve the management of pulmonary diseases [4, 5].

Specific problems in children

Most pediatric Nuclear Medicine examinations have been carried out in general departments. Nevertheless, a specific approach is necessary for children. Most pediatric studies should be performed the same day. The time required for pediatric investigation is usually twice the time needed for a similar study in an adult. Premedication is usually not required as long as enough time is devoted to obtaining the child's confidence. Younger patients (less than one year of age) can be immobilized using sand bags or an inflatable air mattress. A team particularly specialized in specific pediatric problems is highly desirable.

Radiation doses in children

Nuclear Medecine physicians and pediatricians have often been reluctant to use radionuclides in children. The main reason appears to be poor knowledge of the radiation doses involved and of the potential hazards (table 1).

The Pediatric Task Group of the European Association of Nuclear Medicine recently suggested a method to estimate the amounts of radio-pharmaceuticals to be administered at various ages [6]. Although more studies are still needed [7], the delivered radiation dose remains low enough to allow such investigations in children [6]. Moreover, the amount of radioactivity administered should not drop too far in order to avoid poor quality images. Minimal values have been published [6].

Methods

Pediatric and adult scintigraphic procedures are not dissimilar: combined ventilation and perfusion studies are required. Regional function abnormalities usually result in local scintigraphic abnormalities of the ventilation-perfusion ratio (V/Q). At least 100 kcounts per view in ventilation and 200 kcounts in perfusion are required.The accuracy of radionuclide studies is improved if correlated with chest X-ray.

The effect of posture on both ventilation and perfusion images has been recognized for a long time. Since consistency is required to compare sequential studies in children, inspiration of the radionuclide, injection and scans must always be carried out in the supine position.

Ventilation studies

^{81m}Kr gas ventilation studies can be carried out even without the cooperation of the child. The very short

Table 1. Radiation doses to the lungs, ovaries and testes for several pulmonary nuclear medicine procedures in children

Study	Radiopharmaceutical Type	Activity (MBq)	Radiation dose Lungs*	µGy/MBq Ovaries/testes**
Perfusion	^{99m}Tc -MAA	10-75	850-250 (0-2 y.) 150-70 (5-15 y.)	5/1.35
	^{133}Xe solution	37	5	0.5/0.125
Ventilation	^{81m}Kr	75-150	0.25	0.01/0.01
	Technegas	7-50***	125	0.25/0.125
	^{133}Xe gas	75-200	3	0.25/0.25

* Chest X-ray (anterior +lateral view)= 1000 µGy; ** chest X-ray (anterior +lateral view)= 2.5/1.25 µGy; *** depending on the inspiration quality

half-life (T1/2 = 13 sec) may allow repeat studies since the radiation dose is low. However, this radiopharmaceutical is not readily available. In addition, because of the high ventilation turnover, the images may reflect lung volume rather than ventilation.

^{133}Xe gas can be used in a cooperative child. Regional Washout and Trapping can be evaluated only with xenon-133. On the other hand, the images are of poor quality and no more than 2 views can usually be recorded for a reasonable irradiation. Therefore, accurate V/Q comparison is difficult. In addition, good cooperation of the child is required. For all these reasons, 133Xe cannot be used in babies or small children.

"Solid (Technegas (R)) or liquid drop aerosols" labeled with technetium-99m may be of value in pediatrics. Only moderate cooperation is required from the child and this radiopharmaceutical is readily available; a full series of images (including anterior, posterior, right and left posterior oblique views) can always be recorded even in neonates. However, no kinetic information regarding regional ventilation function is obtained.

Perfusion studies

Perfusion studies are not dissimilar to those carried out in adults. Albumin macroaggregates or microspheres labeled with Technetium-99m are administered intravenously. The number of albumin particles should not exceed 100,000. Albumin cannot be used when a major right to left shunt is suspected (lung or cardiac congenital abnormalities); in such cases, ^{133}Xe in saline solution must be used.

Nuclear medicine (pulmonary) procedures in children

Both ventilation and perfusion studies are usually gathered within a single procedure. The order depends on the clinical problems and the physical characteristics of the radionuclides. If the same radionuclide (e.g. ^{99m}Tc) is used for both studies, it is necessary to increase the radioactivity (and thus the radiation dose) injected for the perfusion study, so that a V/Q count ratio above 4 is obtained.

Scintigraphic maturation patterns

Scintigraphic patterns of lung maturation in normal neonates are poorly documented. When carried out in neonates, ^{81m}Kr ventilation study may occasionally show segmental defects without clear physiological explanation.

Scintigraphic imaging in pediatric pulmonary pathology

Foreign body inhalation

Lung scintigraphy is useful when a suspicion of foreign body inhalation persists in spite of a normal chest X-ray. In such cases, ventilation or perfusion scintigraphy may show a photopenic segmental or lobar defect and then be a guide for subsequent endoscopy. Functional recovery can be scintigraphically established, or disproved if fragmentation of the foreign body occurs during extraction.

Abnormalities persisting after 6 months strongly suggest sequelae. Regional lung function in subsequent chronic lesions such as granulomas and bronchiectasis may be scintigraphically assessed and followed up.

Primary bronchiectasis and sequelae of infectious disease

If bronchiectasis is suspected in a child in spite of a normal chest radiograph, lung scintigraphy may be helpful in children as screening before bronchography (more invasive) or before CT (involving a higher hazard). However in 5% of patients with bronchiectasis, both chest X-ray and lung scintigraphy are normal. Repeat scintigraphy may assess the evolution of the regional dysfunction in these patients.

Pulmonary embolism

The diagnosis of pulmonary embolism in children is not more difficult than in adults as long as a ventilation study is performed. Nevertheless, clinical, biological and radiological data are necessary to avoid misinterpretation: congenital lung and heart abnormalities (see below), arterial pulmonary hypertension or abnormal pulmonary venous return may result in a V/Q mismatch.

One particular point is the acute chest syndrome in children with sickle cell disease: the challenge for lung scintigraphy is to distinguish between pulmonary infarction and infection. Usually, more abnormalities are seen on the perfusion images in lung infarction (usual V/Q mismatch). Ventilation defects are predominant in pneumonia (reverse Q/V mismatch).

Congenital lung and heart abnormalities

Pulmonary ventilation and perfusion abnormalities and V/Q mismatch or imbalance may be related to a large range of abnormal developments of the respiratory and vascular components such as stenosis, agenesis of a branch of the pulmonary artery, communication between aorta and right pulmonary artery, or congenital heart disease such as the Tetralogy of Fallot.

Pulmonary sequestrations are vascularized through the systemic circulation, which may be assessed by radionuclide angiography using pertechnetate 99mTc. On perfusion study with ^{99m}Tc-MAA, there is evidence of poor uptake in the sequestered area. The ventilation study may be normal.

Asthma

Lung scintigraphy may assess a focal etiology in the early management of an asthmatic syndrome. Scintigraphy is only reliable when performed between crises.

Mucoviscidosis

The usefulness of muco ciliary clearance with serum albumin labeled with technetium-99m study in patients with mucoviscidosis has been emphasized in adults. Very few studies have been described in children.

Chest tumors

As in adults, enlarged tumoral lymph nodes may lead to the compression of a bronchus or a branch of the pulmonary artery, resulting in ventilation or perfusion abnormalities.

In lymphomas, ^{67}Ga scintigraphy provides the same information as in adults.

Calcified pulmonary metastases in patients with osteogenic sarcoma may be seen on 99mTc-HMDP bone scan. However, CT seems to be more accurate in such cases. Pulmonary metastases are exceptional in neuroblastomas, but may be scintigraphically assessed using meta-iodobenzylguanidine (MIBG) labeled with radioactive iodine.

Scoliosis

The functional impairment subsequent to severe scoliosis may be assessed by ^{133}Xe ventilation studies and help the surgical decision.

Recurrent chest disease and gastro-esophageal reflux

Some cases of asthma or recurrent lung infection may be related to gastro-esophageal reflux. Pulmonary aspiration can be detected on delayed thoracic images of ^{99m}Tc-sulphur colloid scan. In younger patients, the radiopharmaceutical may be mixed with milk ("milk scan"). The radiation hazard remains within reasonable limits. Unfortunately, the sensitivity is low, since the probability that a pulmonary aspiration might occur during the scintigraphic examination is also low. Therefore, direct evidence is rarely observed even in patients selected on the basis of respiratory symptoms. Nevertheless, it is not unusual for gastro-esophageal scintigraphy to be the only evidence of pulmonary aspiration and it usually shows abnormal esophageal reflux. Moreover, in view of the low radiation hazard, it may be repeated in order to assess the efficiency of an antireflux treatment. Quantitative evaluation of pulmonary aspiration may be more sensitive and has been proposed with additional radioactive measurements of bronchial material in artificially ventilated infants.

Conclusion

Pulmonary scintigraphy is the best noninvasive method to evaluate regional ventilation and perfusion in pediatrics. With minimal radiation, it can improve the management of many pulmonary diseases.

References

1. Gordon I, Helms P, Fazio F (1981) Clinical applications of radionuclide lung scanning in infants and children. Br J Radiol 54 : 576-585
2. Guillet J, Basse-Cathalinat B, Christophe E, Saudubray F (1983) Scintigraphie pulmonaire de ventilation et de perfusion en pathologie respiratoire infantile. Ann Pédiat 30, 4 : 247-255
3. Piepsz A, Gordon I, Hahn K (1991) Paediatric nuclear medicine. Eur J Nucl Med 18 : 41-66
4. Ablin D, Newell J (1987) Diagnostic Imaging for Evaluation of the Pediatric Chest. Clin Chest Med 8, 4 : 641-660
5. Ciofetta G, Gordon I, Piepsz A (1988) Clinical applications of nuclear medicine. Arch Dis Child 63 : 321-328
6. Paediatric Task Group European Association Nuclear Medicine Members (1990) A radiopharmaceuticals schedule for imaging in paediatrics. Eur J Nucl Med 17 : 127-129
7. Mountford PJ (1991) Radiation protection for the parent and child in diagnostic nuclear medicine. Eur J Nucl Med 18 : 940-943

Optimization of aerosol administration by nuclear medicine techniques

P Diot and G Smaldone

The aerosol is becoming a more and more common way of administering drugs. It was used for a long time in asthmatic patients to administer beta 2, anticholinergics, cromones and, more recently, steroids. Pentamidine for HIV patients for the prophylaxis of Pneumocystis carinii pneumonia, and antibiotics such as colimycin or tobramycin for cystic fibrosis patients infected with Pseudomonas aeruginosa, are administered as aerosols. Aerosols of amiloride, DNase and nucleotides appear to be of value in cystic fibrosis patients in order to fight against rheological alterations of the mucous. Studies are in progress to define the place of cyclosporin aerosols after pulmonary transplantation. Gene therapy, if clinically relevant, will be administered as an aerosol in patients with emphysema or cystic fibrosis.

Antiasthmatic drugs such as MDI or dry powdered inhalers are available. Most of the other drugs have yet to be administered using an ultrasonic or jet nebulizer. Since the beginning of the AIDS epidemic, Pneumocystis carinii pneumonia prophylaxis has required the definition of optimal conditions for nebulization of pentamidine. This has focused on the necessity to standardize as much as possible the characterization and kinetic studies of aerosols. It was shown, for example, that hydrophilic drugs can be influenced in terms of MMAD, and therefore bronchial kinetics, by the high humidity degree of the respiratory tract. It appears therefore that the MMAD is not constant for a known nebulizer and in fact also depends on the physico-chemical properties of the drug to be nebulized. Moreover the kinetics of the drug have ideally to be assessed in vivo to take into account all the parameters related to the specific physiological and pathophysiological conditions of an individual patient with a known disease.

Nuclear medicine plays a crucial role in this context. When strict methodological conditions are applied, the nuclear medicine approach has proved to be relevant for the assessment of both particle size distribution and in vivo kinetics studies.

Methodology

The use of isotopic methods for characterization and kinetic analysis of aerosols necessitates strict respect of methodological rules and definition of parameters to be assessed.

A methodological understanding is necessary when using radioactivity as a measurement technique.

The common aim is to assess the kinetics of a certain mass of molecule M by counting a certain number of counts per minute obtained from a radio isotope I* (most often a gamma-emitter) by using a gamma camera or a gamma counter.

Nevertheless, it can never be considered that mass of M can simply be appreciated by counts per minute (CPM) obtained from I*. In fact the relationship between these 2 parameters can be formalized as follows:

$$\text{x mg M} \overset{(1)}{\longleftrightarrow} \text{X MBq I*} \overset{(2)}{\longleftrightarrow} \text{X' DPM} \overset{(3)}{\longleftrightarrow} \text{X'' CPM}$$

Each of these 3 mathematical relationships has to be taken into account to ensure the relevance of the isotopic approach. None of them corresponds to an

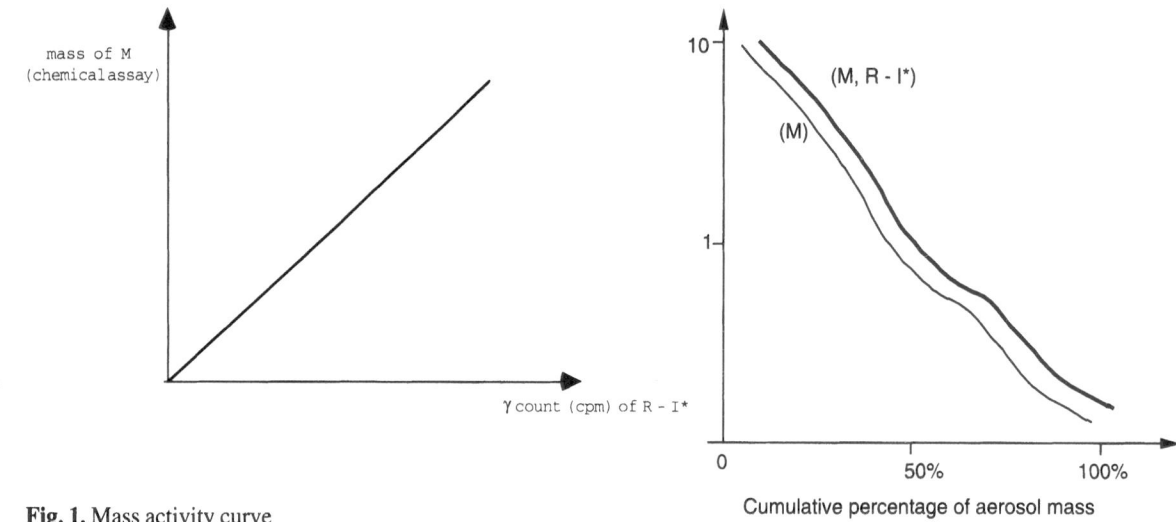

Fig. 1. Mass activity curve

Fig. 2. Comparison of particle size distribution of M and (M, R-I*)

equation but to a relationship based on a converting coefficient which can depend upon technical, physical or biochemical specificities.

Relationship (3) is essential from a technical point of view. This expresses the relationship between the physical phenomenon of radioactive degradation (DPM) and its count (CPM) based on technical equipment. This means that the counting material has to be regularly calibrated with different known radioactivity doses. This is the usual quality control of any measurement method and appears to be particularly important when considering the isotopic approach. It is indeed well known that the count ratio varies from one material to another and, for a known material, from one time or radioactivity dose to another.

Relationship (2) corresponds to the well known physical constant which establishes that 1 Bq = 60 DPM.

Relationship (1) is actually the one to be established.

To establish relationship (1), the molecule to be studied can be labeled either directly or indirectly, taking into account relationships (2) and (3).

The direct method consists of labeling the drug itself. The technique is very well known for proteins and widely used for labeling albumin for example [1].This is much more difficult for complex molecules such as drugs and requires a very specialized radio-chemical approach. The radiolabeling must involve the pharmacologically active principle itself and not the excipient. Nevertheless kinetics study of the aerosolized drug must involve the active radiolabeled principle mixed with its excipient to reproduce the actual conditions of treatment. The excipient can influence the aerosol kinetics by its own physico-chemical properties. It was clearly demonstrated for example that oleic acid mixed with beclomethasone can induce cough and even bronchospasm and therefore can alter the bronchial kinetics of the inhaled steroid. Quality controls of the labeling must be performed in vitro by radiochromatography. Stability of labeling must be assessed in vivo, ideally after inhalation, taking into account the fact that the physical mechanism involved to nebulize the solution (ultrasound or compressed gas) could dissociate the labeling. When ^{99m}Tc is used, the absence of thyroid fixation must at least be assessed.

Much easier in terms of the physico-chemical process is the indirect approach. When applied under the control of strict methodology, this approach has proved to be fully relevant with many molecules. This methodology was defined step by step since new interest was focused on pentamidine aerosols by the AIDS epidemic. This consists of mixing the molecule to be studied with a radio-labeled reference, most often albumin or colloid. As stated above, methods to label such proteins, especially with ^{99m}Tc, have been precisely described and are routinely applied to clinical applications. Therefore similar procedures, even if used as a research tool, do not require any special quality control. The problem is to establish first that both the molecule (M) to be studied and the radio-labeled reference (R-I*) have the same kinetics characteristics and second that mixing M with R-I* does not modify particle size distribution.

Similarity of kinetics of M and R-I* is assessed by determining a mass activity curve. This is easily performed by the cascade impaction method. It consists of sampling the aerosol by range of size on glass slides covering superimposed cylinders, all of them being centered by a hole of decreasing diameter. On each of the slides, there is impaction of part of the aerosol made of particles characterized by an aerodynamic diameter greater than the diameter of the considered hole. Impacted fractions on each of the slides can be separately diluted to measure the mass of M of each of the samples on the one hand and radioactivity corresponding to R-I* on the other hand. It is then easy to draw a graph with radioactivity on the horizontal axis and mass on the vertical axis. Distribution of points along a bisective line proves the relevance of R-I* measurement to assess the kinetics of M (fig. 1).

This approach obviously requires a method for the measurement of M mass, which is most often based on high purity liquid chromatography methods (HPLC) and precise calibration of the gamma-counter.

Cascade impaction is also the recommended method to study the particle size distribution of aerosols. It consists of measuring cumulative percentage of aerosol impacted on each of the slides from the greatest to the smallest aerodynamic diameter for both M aerosol (HPLC method) and M, R-I* aerosol (gamma-counting or HPLC method). If M and R-I* have the same particle size distribution, in vivo kinetics studies of M, R-I* by isotopic method are relevant to assess the kinetics of the actual M aerosol (fig. 2).

Applications

As described above, the isotopic approach is basically involved in the cascade impaction method. Nevertheless MMAD and σg result from bench studies and do not necessarily reflect what occurs in vivo. Hydrophylic or electric charges for example can influence the kinetics of the aerosol which can differ from the kinetics expected when taking into account only MMAD. Therefore intra-respiratory kinetics of aerosols and other important parameters referring to the performance of nebulizers have obviously to be assessed in vivo in the actual conditions of treatment. Figures 3 and 4 show intrathoracic deposition of directly labeled pentamidine obtained in 2 patients by using the same ultrasonic nebulizer. Pulmonary deposition is obviously much more homogeneous and peripheral in the figure 3 than in the figure 4.

Smaldone [2,3] described in detail methods for measuring different parts of aerosols defined as follows: The inhaled fraction is the actual part of aerosol available for inhalation. In view of the remaining part of the solution in the device at the end of inhalation on the one hand, and of the leakage on the other, the inhaled fraction is always more or less different from the dose deposited in the nebulizer. The deposited fraction is the part of the inhaled aerosol which remains in the respiratory tract. The therapeutic efficacy of an inhaled drug depends upon the deposited fraction and its precise distribution. The exhaled fraction is the part of the inhaled aerosol which is exhaled and may be of no therapeutic value. Figure 5 represents two complementary experimental maneuvers to assess the different fractions.

On the left maneuver, a filter is placed between the patient's mouth and the inspiratory line of the nebulizer. A second filter is placed at the outgang of the expiratory line. In such conditions both the inhaled fraction and leakage can be separately determined.

The inspiratory filter recovers the whole part of the aerosol available for inhalation, i.e. the inhaled fraction. Taking into account that this "theoretically" inhaled fraction is fully and definitively trapped in the inspiratory filter, radio-activity trapped in the expiratory filter strictly corresponds to the leakage. As shown in the right maneuver, suppression of the inspiratory filter makes possible the individualization of 2 more fractions that are the deposited fraction and the exhaled fraction. Indeed, the deposited fraction can be determined by counting the radio-activity present in the thoracic area in the precise methodological conditions described above. This deposited fraction results from subtraction of the exhaled fraction from the inhaled fraction. In such experimental conditions, the expiratory filter activity corresponds to the addition of the leakage, which is a characteristic of the nebulizer and remains whatever the experimental conditions, and the exhaled fraction. Therefore the exhaled fraction can be determined by the subtraction of leakage (as assessed in the first experimental conditions) from the addition of leakage and exhaled fraction (as assessed by the second experimental conditions).

Besides this basic characterization of different fractions of aerosol, nuclear medicine principles of image processing can be applied for intra-respiratory kinetics analysis of the drug. The anatomic site of deposition of the aerosol can be characterized by defining regions of interest on central and peripheral parts of the lungs. This was of particular interest to

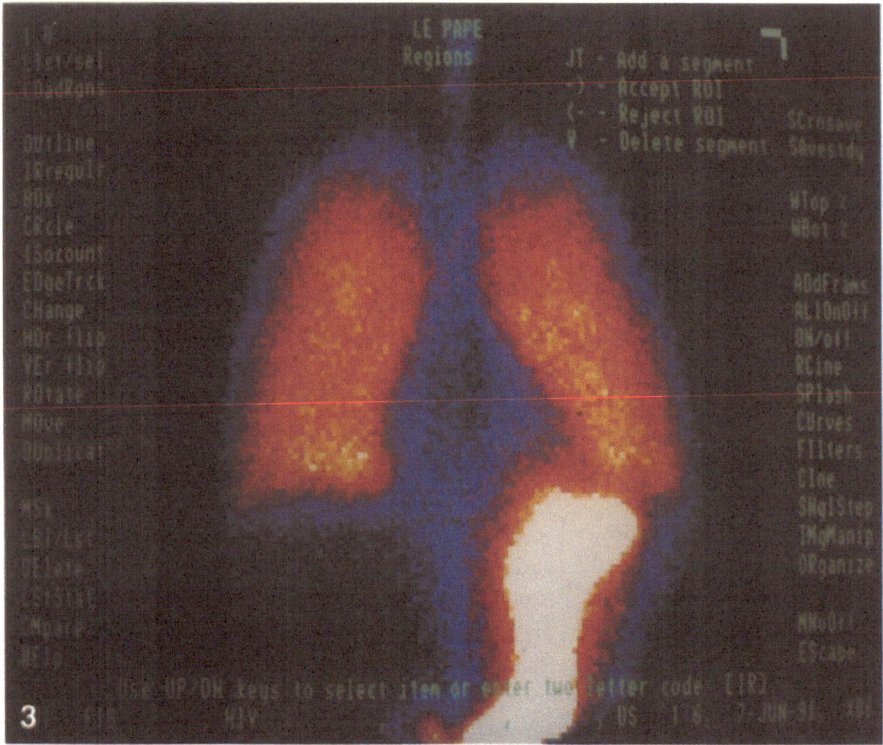

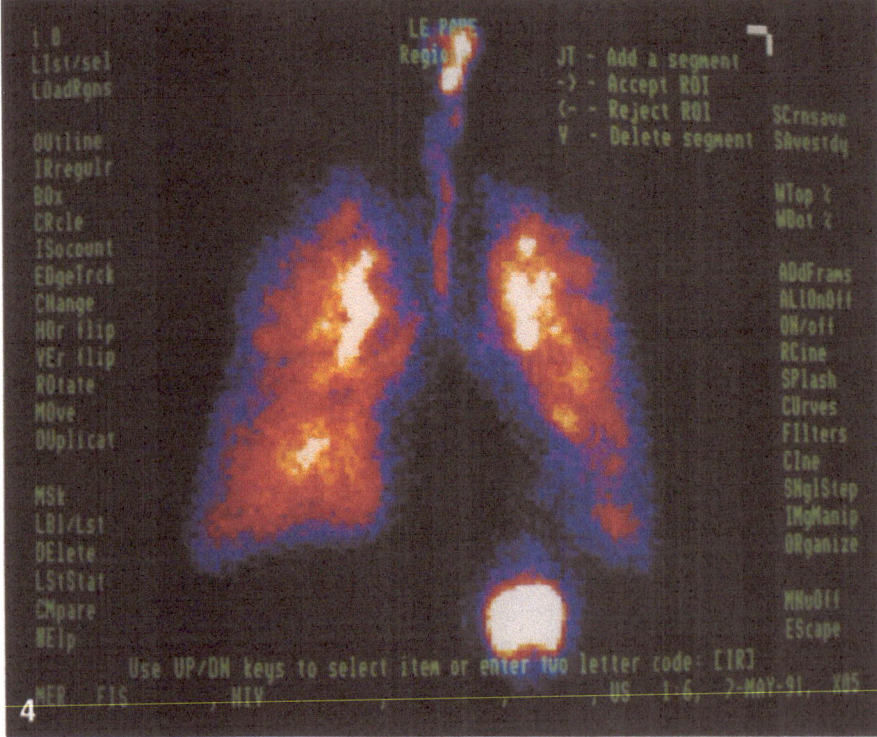

Figs. 3, 4. Pulmonary deposition of directly ^{99m}Tc labeled pentamidine in 2 different patients using the same ultrasonic nebuli-zer (Fisoneb®, Fisons, France). Pulmonary deposition is much more homogeneous and peripheral in the patient represented on the figure 3 than in the patient represented on the figure 4

Inhaled fraction

leakage

Exhaled fraction - leakage

deposited fraction

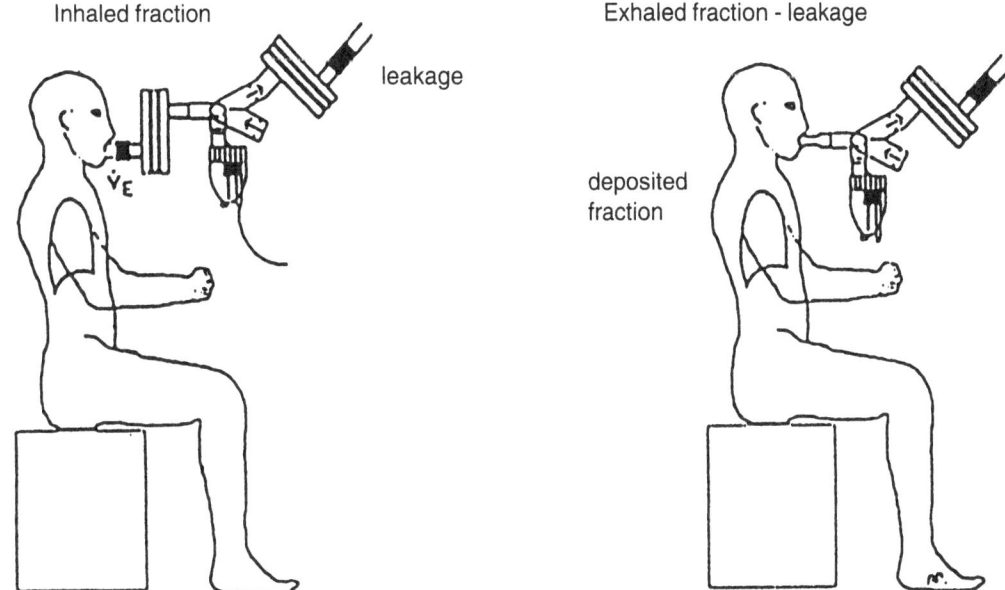

Fig. 5. Two complementary experiments to assess the different parts of the aerosol

define recommendations for administration of aerosolized pentamidine in HIV patients for example. Moreover, systemic absorption or muco-ciliary clearance can be studied according to methods described in the specific chapter.

Therefore, nuclear medicine appears to be a major tool for the study and improvement of aerosoltherapy. There is no doubt that many studies currently in progress in this field will have major practical implications for treatment of respiratory diseases, and maybe some extra-respiratory diseases, in the near future.

References

1. Lin MS, Winchell HS, Shipley BA (1971) Use of Fe (II) or Sn (II) alone for technétium labeling of albumin. J Nucl Med 12 : 204-211

2. Smaldone GC, Fuhrer J, Steigbigel RT, Mc Peck M (1991) Factors determining pulmonary deposition of aero-solized pentamidine in patients with human immunodefi-ciency virus infection. Am Rev Respir Dis 143 : 727-737

3. Smaldone GC (1991) Drug delivery via aérosol systems : concept of "aerosol inhaled". J Aerosol Med 4 : 229-235

Index

A

Acquisition 10, 11, 33, 41, 55, 73, 83, 84, 111
Adenopathy 59, 62, 64, 65, 101
Aerosol 1, 11-13, 18-21, 26, 27,
    31-34, 37, 43, 44, 49, 50, 54, 55, 73,
    84, 100, 101, 103, 114, 117-119, 121
Alveolar Hemorrhage 67, 69, 78
Alveolitis 14, 30, 57, 64, 67, 68, 71,
    72, 75, 98, 100, 101, 103, 105
Asbestosis 58-59, 71

B, C

Bronchiolitis 67, 69-70, 78, 96
Connective 14, 57, 67, 69

D

Diffusion 11, 12, 15, 17, 18, 31, 32, 75, 80
Dosimetry 29, 39, 42, 91
DTPA 26, 27, 30-32, 41-43,
    49-51, 55, 67, 71, 75, 102, 103

F, G

Fibrosis 14, 16, 17, 29, 30, 36,
    57-60, 65-72, 75, 77, 108, 117
Gallium 12, 27-29, 37, 43, 60, 61, 65, 67,
    73-75, 77, 82, 84, 95-101, 103-105

H

Histiocytosis X 57-60, 65
HIV 75, 95-97, 99-103, 105, 117, 121
Hypersensitivity pneumonitis 58-60, 71

I

Immunoscintigraphy 41-43, 80-83, 85-87, 92
Indium 12, 99
Interstitial 14, 17, 30, 31, 57-61, 63, 65,
    67-75, 77, 78, 96, 98, 99, 101, 105
Iodine 115
Isotopes 5, 11, 32, 39, 42, 80, 95, 117

K

Kaposi 75, 95-96, 98, 99, 103
Krypton 12, 26

L

Lung cancer 3, 29, 53-55, 79-82, 85, 87
Lymphocyte 14, 15, 57, 59-61, 65, 67, 69,
    74, 75, 98, 101
Lymphoma 29, 37, 69, 70, 75, 82, 96, 98-100, 115

M

Macro-aggregates 47

Macrophage 1, 14-15, 57, 59, 61, 69,
                               72-73, 78, 80, 84, 85, 87, 101
MIBG 12, 40-43, 85-87, 115
Mucociliary clearance 15, 32, 34-36, 107-108
Mucoviscidosis 36, 115

P

Perfusion 1, 3, 9-12, 17, 18, 23-27, 32,
                               37, 41-43, 45-51, 53-56, 113-116
Pneumoconiosis 30, 59, 70,71, 75, 78, 89
Pneumocystis 30, 75, 95-98, 100, 102-105, 117
Polynuclear 12, 41
Pulmonary embolism 1, 3, 23, 25, 37, 39,
                                                45-51, 96, 115
Pulmonary infiltrate with eosinophilia 66

R

Radioactivity 7-9, 11, 27, 31, 32, 34, 40, 42, 49,
                               81, 82, 100, 109, 113, 114, 117-119
Radiopharmaceuticals 1, 11, 12,
                                     29, 39-42, 85, 93, 113-116

Reflux 108, 109, 115, 116

S

Sarcoidosis 17, 30, 57-65, 71, 73-75, 77, 78, 82, 89
SMS 12, 40, 85-86

T

Technegas 26, 27, 37, 50, 114
Technetium 26, 27, 39

V

Venticis 26, 55
Ventilation 1, 3, 9-13, 15, 17, 18, 23,
                                     24, 26, 32, 37, 40-43, 45,
                                     48-51, 53-56, 107, 113-116

W, X

Wegener 66
Xenon 8-10, 12, 24, 26

Publishing, cover: François Leprince, Paris